The Natural Hormone Makeover

10 Steps to Rejuvenate Your Health and Rediscover Your Inner Glow

Phuli Cohan, M.D.

WILEY

John Wiley & Sons, Inc.

Published by John Wiley & Sons, Inc., Hoboken, New Jersey
Published simultaneously in Canada

Illustrations by Robert Romano; copyright © 2008 by Phuli Cohan

No part of this publication may be reproduced, stored in a retrieval system, or transmitted in any form or by any means, electronic, mechanical, photocopying, recording, scanning, or otherwise, except as permitted under Section 107 or 108 of the 1976 United States Copyright Act, without either the prior written permission of the Publisher, or authorization through payment of the appropriate per-copy fee to the Copyright Clearance Center, 222 Rosewood Drive, Danvers, MA 01923, (978) 750-8400, fax (978) 646-8600, or on the web at www.copyright.com. Requests to the Publisher for permission should be addressed to the Permissions Department, John Wiley & Sons, Inc., 111 River Street, Hoboken, NJ 07030, (201) 748-6011, fax (201) 748-6008, or online at http://www.wiley.com/go/permissions.

The information contained in this book is not intended to serve as a replacement for professional medical advice. Any use of the information in this book is at the reader's discretion. The author and the publisher specifically disclaim any and all liability arising directly or indirectly from the use or application of any information contained in this book. A health care professional should be consulted regarding your specific situation.

For general information about our other products and services, please contact our Customer Care Department within the United States at (800) 762-2974, outside the United States at (317) 572-3993 or fax (317) 572-4002.

Wiley also publishes its books in a variety of electronic formats. Some content that appears in print may not be available in electronic books. For more information about Wiley products, visit our web site at www.wiley.com.

Library of Congress Cataloging-in-Publication Data:

Cohan, Phuli, date.
  The natural hormone makeover : 10 steps to rejuvenate your health and rediscover your inner glow / Phuli Cohan.
     p. cm.
  Includes bibliographical references and index.
  ISBN 978-0-471-74484-9 (cloth)
  1. Hormone therapy—Popular works. 2. Women—Health and hygiene. 3. Endocrine gynecology—Popular works. 4. Rejuvenation. I. Title.
  RM286.C64 2008
  615'.36—dc22

                                                          2007044824

Printed in the United States of America

10 9 8 7 6 5 4 3 2 1

To my teachers in Asia, Australasia, Europe, and the United States who taught me to bring common sense and balance to medicine

To my patients, whose success using natural hormones compelled me to write this book

To the healthcare professionals responsible for the Women's Health Initiative Study, which helped bring an end to the "one pill for all" treatment of women. Much of the debate about the safe use of hormones started with their efforts.

To my husband: this book could not have been written without your unwavering support and love. You make it all possible.

Contents

Introduction — 1

1 Understanding Health and Hormones — 13

2 The Ten-Step Hormone Makeover — 21

3 Hormone Safety and Metabolism — 29

4 Hormones and a Healthy Lifestyle — 57

5 Know Your Symptoms — 81

6 Recommended Tests — 99

7 How to Find the Right Doctor and Support Team — 109

8 Sex Hormones Part 1: Perimenopause and Progesterone — 115

9 Sex Hormones Part 2: Using Natural Bioidentical Estrogen and Testosterone — 137

10 Adrenal and Thyroid Hormones — 177

11 Sleep Hormones — 219

12 Growth Hormone — 233

Conclusion — 241

Appendix A: Symptoms of Low Hormones   245

Appendix B: Symptoms of Hormone Excess   251

References   255

Suggested Readings   273

Index   274

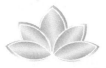

Introduction

I have been described as a "naturalist" physician, and that's probably as close as you can get to explaining what I do. After graduating from Brown University Medical School in 1982, I was excited but also somewhat dismayed. Despite top-notch medical training, something was missing. Medicine seemed impersonal, overly technical, and disjointed. Systems and specialties were taught separately; pieces weren't fully connected. The cardiovascular system was never linked to moods, yet I noticed that most people who had suffered a heart attack often had upsetting dreams or felt depressed, more so than with other illnesses. No one seemed to notice how the menstrual cycle affected a woman's bowels, yet most women, when asked, will tell you that they do often change. Nutrition was discussed in terms of calories or "exchanges" without any connection to hormones or neurotransmitters, which are made from proteins and are carefully regulated by our vitamins and minerals. Physical signs that people noticed about themselves, such as their tongue coating or the quality of their skin, nails, and hair, were largely overlooked.

So after leaving medical school, I deferred my internship for a year and traveled to India and Sri Lanka, where I worked alongside Ayurvedic doctors, herbalists, and homeopaths. In the East, it is not uncommon for such alternative doctors to work alongside physicians. I watched as pulses and tongues were examined and dreams and fears were carefully discussed. I came to appreciate a larger picture of health and disease. Sure, medications are important, but in the East attention to symptoms is most important. I never heard a homeopath or Ayurvedic doctor say, "You're fine, there is nothing wrong with you, these symptoms are just in your mind," or "You are simply depressed or overworked." Each symptom, no matter how minute, was noted and considered as a powerful clue to the patient's problem.

I returned to the United States in 1983 to begin an exciting internship in family medicine. I delivered more than a hundred babies and performed dozens of C-sections and thoroughly loved my work, but I was still restless. I had a professor in medical school from New Zealand, and I remembered how he had meticulously listened to the heart only after carefully considering the shape of the fingers and the quality of the hair and skin, all signs of how the blood from the heart was truly acting. That particular piece of my medical school training left a lasting impression. So after my first internship I signed on for a second one—another year of sleepless nights, this time halfway around the world in New Zealand, where my professor had come from and where there were but two CAT scans for the entire population of over 3.5 million people. You had no hope of getting your patient to a scan unless you could precisely determine, from your astute physical exam, where exactly in the brain the suspected lesion lay. It was training that emphasized physical signs and symptoms, in lieu of the latest diagnostic machine.

After a year in rural New Zealand, I continued my training at Auckland University studying geriatrics, the medicine of aging, the inevitable condition we all face. It was in this setting in 1984 that I met a professor of rheumatology. Dr. Gerald Gibb had been one of a handful of noted physicians selected by the World Health Organization to visit China when foreigners were first permitted inside the Great Wall. He initiated me into the practice of acupuncture and gave me a taste of

Chinese medical theory. For the first time, I began to understand the connection between emotions, symptoms, diet, and the environment. For the Chinese, there was no such thing as disease, there was simply balance and imbalance. You were either in balance or out of balance.

At last, Chinese medicine satisfied my medical curiosity and opened me to a world that drew together all aspects of the human experience. The Chinese system of diagnosis is symptom-based, not system-based. A system is normally in balance; symptoms signal an imbalance, either a deficiency or an excess, either too much cold or too much heat, for example. Symptoms hold the key to restoring balance. How a person sleeps, thinks, speaks, menstruates, and dreams provides the clues to the underlying problem. There is no separation between emotional and physical symptoms. Symptoms are seen as a continuum from healthy to unwell. Disease as we see it is merely the end product of prolonged imbalance and deficiency of nutrients and energy. In Chinese medicine, age is seen as a gradual decline in kidney *qi* (pronounced "chee") and, though inevitable, this decline can actually be made more gradual and much more comfortable.

With great enthusiasm I began using acupuncture on my geriatric patients. I noticed that my stroke patients could move more freely and that their moods and bowels improved. I began treating patients who had heart problems and saw that by inserting an acupuncture needle in their arm (which at one time was embryologically linked to their heart), I could ease their heart palpitations and even calm their racing minds. This fascinated me because I remembered the Chinese saying "The heart rules the mind."

After three years in New Zealand, I left to complete the U.S. acupuncture training for physicians at UCLA in 1989, and then worked for three years at a clinic in Hawaii. I used acupuncture and herbs, as well as traditional Western medicine, to treat whatever ailments walked through the door. The local Hawaiian kahunas, or healers, were similar to the Chinese—always considering the emotional and spiritual beliefs of their patients, using deep massage and herbs to bring people into balance. This experience drove me to want more traditional training in Chinese medicine, not just the rote map of acupuncture points that Western doctors had given me.

So I traveled to Australia to complete my training in emergency medicine and, more important to me, to study Chinese gynecology with Dr. Steven Clavey. Each week I worked alongside him in conjunction with leading gynecologists in Melbourne, to treat and study women with pelvic pain caused by endometriosis. I saw that after their surgery, if herbs and acupuncture were used, their symptoms were less likely to recur. Dr. Clavey taught me about the ebb and flow of women's hormones with a traditional Chinese perspective. We worked to improve women's "liver flow" (or hormone breakdown, as I saw it). I burned mugwort (an ancient herb used in Chinese medicine to warm and nourish the meridians) on their bellies and discussed imbalances in their diets and lifestyles. It became clear to me that these ancient healing systems had a place in the modern world and that we Western physicians had much to learn from their study. I saw that our science was complementary and could explain, biochemically, their poetic beliefs.

Chinese medicine recognizes that as we age, we need to be nourished and fortified with "tonics." It is this notion that brought me to my understanding of hormonal health. I have learned that you can use hormones as tonics to restore the deficiencies of age and to lessen the effects of stress, illness, and poor lifestyle.

I now run a holistic medical practice near Boston, Massachusetts, merging Eastern and Western medicine. Using both systems, I treat women to alleviate their many painful and unpleasant symptoms of perimenopause and menopause. Whereas Western medicine alone has afforded them no relief, I spend much of my time explaining to my patients how hormones can be used safely, and I spend too much time helping them make sense of the myriad of confusing and often terrifying headlines about hormones, menopause, and disease. That's why I wrote this book.

Medical studies are usually looking for that one cure-all pill for the masses, and doctors too often practice McMedicine, an all-for-one and one-pill-for-all approach. When I graduated from medical school in 1982, all menopausal women were told to take horse estrogen and synthetic progesterone. Then, twenty years later, after the Women's Health Initiative (WHI) study was released in 2002, a panic swept through the medical community, and millions of women were abruptly taken off their horse hormones, leaving them with no safe alternative treatments for their sometimes unbearable symptoms. Women were told either to "tough it out" or to take antidepressants. They weren't informed about other options, such as low-dose bioidentical hormones, administered via transdermal (skin) creams with individualized dosing, which have been used by European physicians for more than two decades. They weren't told that adrenal hormones such as DHEA or other therapies could support estrogen production and promote deeper sleep, better mood, and more energy, and even enhance their sex drive. Nobody was taking the time to explain the whole picture of how hormones work, and how most breast cancers form.

So here is a point that you will hear me make often as we discuss and simplify some very complicated subjects. *Hormones should be used, and they can be used safely. Using bioidentical estrogen and progesterone in individualized doses, while monitoring hormone metabolites, is safe and may actually lower breast cancer risks as well as the risks of bone disease, dementia, heart disease, and other cancers.* These treatments have spared my patients and me from many of the agonies of perimenopause and menopause, and I know they can do the same for you.

I will also explain the results of the WHI study and other mega-studies that have added confusion to the debate about using hormones. The findings of the WHI study were for the most part predictable, and when you look at them carefully, the results are actually encouraging.

The Natural Hormone Makeover is intended to guide the millions of women who feel lousy and suffer fatigue, headaches, mood swings, heavy bleeds, low sex drive, and sleepless nights. It can also serve as a guide for women of any age suffering from deficiencies or imbalances of hormones. This book will help women to take charge of their own health.

Symptoms are not the enemy to be masked by the latest new drug on the market. We must carefully listen to our symptoms. They are feedback from our body that there is imbalance, deficiency, or injury of some kind. Sure, you may be getting older, but you feel lousy because you are out of balance. By understanding hormonal symptoms, you can learn how to bring hormonal balance back safely. Only then will you enjoy growing older, and have better sex, more energy, and a good night's sleep as you age.

I discovered the world of bioidentical hormones as many people do, after I was burned out, in my forties. A typical overworked and over-stressed professional, I was raised in the heart of the women's liberation era. I believed that I could and should do anything and everything I wanted to do. A family? Of course. A profession? Most definitely. I had worked in emergency medicine, helicopter rescue, and disaster medi-cine, all while studying Chinese medicine and emergency medicine on four continents.

I married when I was forty, and I inherited five stepchildren. They are all wonderful kids, but I wanted a child of my own. A sixth child at the age of forty, with five kids and a full-time job? Why not? Like most overachieving women my age, I was sure I would become pregnant eas-ily, but this was not to be. Years of hard work and lack of sleep had taken a toll on my egg supply. After the emotional roller-coaster ride of infertility treatments, my husband and I opted to adopt a sixth child, a godsend that satisfied my every maternal urge.

At the age of forty-two I had it all—a wonderful family, an exciting career. But I was on the go day and night, and my forty-something body was changing. I began having symptoms that herbs and acupuncture couldn't seem to alter for more than a day or two. Sleep eluded me even though I was bone-tired most nights. Staying asleep also became diffi-cult—3 a.m. and 5 a.m. were my new wake-up times. During the day I started burning out by 4 p.m. and couldn't wait to get home and just put my feet up. I'd fall asleep in movies or at soccer games, and it seemed I was catching a cold from every person I met. My interest in sex was on a downhill slide, and if someone crossed me the wrong way—watch out! I became moody, and PMS, which had never been a big issue, was unbearable. I found myself losing my temper with the very people I loved the most.

I knew I was off—hormonally off—but I didn't know what to do. I had always been anti–hormone replacement. After all, I had studied Chinese medicine in order to avoid prescribing drugs and synthetic hormones. Birth control pills in the past had left me feeling nearly sui-cidal, and I saw that synthetic hormones were constantly causing unpleasant side effects in my patients. When I prescribed birth control pills to alleviate the symptoms of menopause in them, new symptoms would erupt, such as breast swelling, headaches, bloating, mood swings, and worst of all, weight gain. I call that "symptom swapping." So I considered what I knew from Chinese medicine.

The Chinese have always emphasized the kidney as a source of energy, necessary for fertility and healthy aging. They view aging and perimenopausal symptoms as "kidney deficiency." Of course, I had learned about the kidney in medical school but not about its relationship to healthy aging. When I learned about the Chinese view in my thirties, I began using Chinese medicine to strengthen my kidneys. I drank foul-tasting Chinese herbs; on my ankles I heated moxa (a Chinese herb that is burned near acupuncture needles to help strengthen the body)—all to improve my kidneys.

I had always believed that whatever Chinese medicine taught, there had to be a Western medical corollary. For example, thousands of years ago, the Chinese believed that the kidney ruled the blood; yet it wasn't until recently that Western medicine discovered the hormone erythropoietin, produced by the kidney, which indeed controls blood cell production and is now used to treat anemia.

So I studied the Chinese kidney, and one day it hit me. The Chinese were not speaking of the kidney organ as understood by Western medicine, they were actually referring to the small adrenal glands lying atop the kidneys. These powerful life-sustaining, hormone-rich glands are our main source of vitality—producing cortisol, aldosterone, pregnenolone, DHEA, and adrenaline. These are all energizing hormones that could in fact enhance our sex drive and fertility, exactly as the Chinese promised. It all fit perfectly. Hormones could be used as tonics to strengthen us.

But women can't take hormones anymore, right? Isn't that what the studies show? Wrong. The studies that have made the headlines are all about *synthetic* hormones, not *natural* hormones. Natural hormones look and feel exactly like the hormones our body produces. In medical school we focused primarily on synthetic hormones. It was, after all, during my training in the 1980s that Premarin (synthetic horse estrogen) was the number-one prescribed drug for women. Now, twenty years later, I learned about adrenal hormones and hormonal "personality" types, like the sexy, exciting feelings that come from estradiol, the confidence-instilling attributes of testosterone, and the calming effects of progesterone. I became familiar with the adrenal hormone

DHEA, the most abundant hormone in our bodies, which improves memory, sex drive, and mood, deepens sleep, and even helps to grow stronger bones.

I learned that the thyroid hormone needs many minerals as well as cortisol and DHEA to become fully active inside our cells. I hadn't fully comprehended that as we age, our adrenal health is vital to produce enough stress and sex hormones to ensure a happy, energetic old age. Understanding hormones and how they interact with one another made sense of both Western and Chinese medicine. I now understood how treating the Chinese kidney (really the adrenal glands) could enhance natural hormone production, and how using bioidentical hormones like a tonic could actually improve long-term health.

In 1998 I attended a five-day natural hormone conference with Dr. Thierry Hertoghe, a leading anti-aging physician from Belgium. He plucked me from the audience as a prime example of forty-something aging. Dr. Hertoghe made sure everyone got a good look at my thinning outer eyebrows, the "gooseflesh" skin of my upper arms, my dry skin, and my slow ankle reflexes (low active thyroid). My sagging cheeks (deficient growth hormone) and reddened eyelids (lack of cortisol) were duly noted, as were my fingernails, which were thin and dry with ridges. Dr. Hertoghe pointed to the wrinkles about my mouth and eyes, consistent with my waning estrogen.

If I could have found a hole, I would have sunk into it. I was embarrassed and horrified but also a bit excited and hopeful. It was like a Chinese diagnosis with a Western slant. It was blood and yin deficiency (the Chinese diagnosis I had been given throughout my thirties) described hormonally, in Western terms. This was the first time that I became aware of just how many symptoms and signs of hormonal deficiency I was exhibiting. At the age of forty-two, I was not just overworked and burned-out, I was experiencing accelerated hormone decline. Even though my weight was stable and my periods were regular, I was hormonally deficient. So I measured the hormone levels in both my blood and urine. The blood tests showed low red blood cell magnesium and low iron stores (low ferritin, but no anemia), low adrenal hormones (low pregnenolone and DHEA), low sex hormones (estrogen and progesterone), and a borderline normal thyroid. The twenty-four-hour urine test showed low levels of growth hormone, cortisol, active thyroid hormone (T3), and aldosterone. I always knew by Chinese standards that I was yin deficient; now I understood why by Western testing. I discovered that I was in fact running at about 50 percent!

This was the beginning for me. I discovered compounding pharmacists in my area (there are over a dozen in Massachusetts). With their help and expertise, I began using natural hormones in small, carefully monitored doses. With just a 5 mg dose of cortisol in the morning, my life began to turn around. I had more constant energy, and my irritability disappeared. Low doses of natural thyroid extract and natural estradiol cream brought my sex drive back up, and aldosterone support improved my stamina. DHEA helped my mood and endurance, and progesterone eased my PMS symptoms. Everything improved except my sleep, which didn't improve fully until I added a growth hormone support.

Over the ensuing years I made lifestyle changes to ensure that my adrenal and thyroid glands stayed healthy. I stopped working overnight shifts and started exercising regularly, eating better, and taking more vacations. I reclaimed myself using natural hormones.

I have been on a natural hormone program for more than eight years and I have entered my fifties feeling better than I did in my thirties.

But it's important to remember that my regimen of pills and creams hasn't stayed the same, and it shouldn't for you, either. Initially when I started on cortisol to support my adrenals, I felt great. After a few months, I noticed that my sleep was less deep. I didn't see this as scary or dangerous; I was happy that I no longer needed cortisol, so I substituted it for a less stimulating adrenal extract for a couple of months. I still had good energy, and my sleep improved immediately. Months later, when my sleep lightened again, I knew to switch to a milder herbal support (*Panax ginseng*) once in the morning, which I still use. Although I no longer use cortisol regularly, I may use it to help me when I am sick or jet-lagged, because I know my cortisol is low.

In addition to supporting my adrenals with cortisol or herbs, I use DHEA (2 to 15 mg/day) intermittently in low doses. After a few months, if I notice any hair thinning or pimples, I take a break from the DHEA and retest. I maintain a DHEA level at midrange for a forty-year-old. My thyroid function improved after I brought my magnesium,

DHEA, and iron up to normal values. I no longer take any thyroid hormones, but I check my levels every year. When I was in my early forties, I used progesterone but I didn't need any estrogen. Then, when I was about forty-eight, I started experiencing headaches and some cramping during my period, symptoms that I had never had before. I knew these were signs of low estradiol. I restarted DHEA (2 mg/day) and estradiol lotion (0.3 mg twice daily on days 1 to 25 of my cycle), and my headaches and cramps stopped. So it's not McMedicine and it's not all-for-one and one-for-all. I have learned to take control of my own health program.

We change. We all change. At different rates, at different times, for different reasons—be they genetics, environment, or lifestyle. Our hormonal and dietary supplements must also change. Too often women are put on medications or hormones—the same dose as everyone else, and their regimen is never changed. Such treatments may work initially, but too often I have seen women coming to my office complaining of weight gain, constant breast tenderness, or insomnia, and no one has measured, monitored, or changed their hormones.

For that matter, most people that I meet have taken the same multivitamin or supplements for years, sometimes decades. That's not a good thing either. Supplements are not meant to be taken continuously, in the same dose. Over time this can have toxic effects on your body. In nature, foods and nutrients vary depending on the season. If our eating habits reflected this, our vitamins and minerals would change seasonally. Chinese medicine uses foods as medicine, guided by the seasons. In the fall and spring, when root vegetables are plentiful, "liver cleansing" is advised. In the summer, berries, which are rich in antioxidants, protect us from the sun's radiation while melons cool us. We tend to ignore our seasonal clues about diet that can help to direct our supplement needs. Western science now supports these ideas, and we are living at a time when all philosophies can be used to complement one another.

To be honest, even with the best hormonal and nutritional supports, aging can be tough. I am fifty years old. I love being fifty, but that sounds so clichéd. I resent all of the books and tapes telling us how great it is to be old, telling us to embrace our inner crone, that fifty is the new thirty. There is a lot of pressure and hype to stay young in our culture, and for some women that's a full-time job. You can easily find yourself obsessing about which exercise program won't flare your lower back, whether high protein and low carbs works for you, and how many days you can safely use a sleep aid.

Keeping up with the news can be overwhelming, too. Am I getting the right Pap smear? When should I get a bone density test? Are mammograms really safe? Is Fosamax the new Prempro? What will they find out about using Fosamax or Actonel for ten years? Lately there have been reports of jawbone necrosis in some women using these drugs—what does that foretell? Do they truly strengthen our bones, or do the bones just look better on a bone density test? Will these medications keep me safe from breaking my soon-to-be-eighty-year-old hip? Premarin was in, and twenty years later it's out; but then again it may be back in, but in little doses. Maybe I should just stay on my antidepressant and forget about everything else.

So which way do you go? Hormones or hot flashes? Whom do you trust these days? Well, I say trust your common sense. Our bodies were not designed to follow trends. What is right for some is not right for others. Don't take medicine for the masses. Listen to your body. Listen to your symptoms. If you are having symptoms, look at what is out of balance and correct that. Be wary of something not fully tested in humans. Don't follow the latest medical trend only to find out in twenty years it wasn't right for you. And don't let media hype steer you away from hormone support. Understand what the studies are really saying. Understand that what works for you some of the time may not work for you all of the time, and what works for someone else might not be right for you.

I have personally used and routinely prescribed every hormone discussed in *The Natural Hormone Makeover*. I can assure you that if you are taking too much cortisol, you will not sleep well. If you do not take enough progesterone or too much estradiol, you will have spotting and tender breasts. If you take too much DHEA, you will get pimples and oily skin and you may even get grumpy. You could get overly opinionated on too much testosterone. On the other hand, if you take no hormones your entire life, you will be more prone to depression, fatigue, low sex drive, and bone loss. You will also have more bad hair days. If you are in your forties or fifties and you choose not to use any hormone support, you will be at increased risk of developing bone fractures, heart disease, colon cancer, and dementia. You will also be more likely to suffer from fatigue, depression, low sex drive, and sleep that is not deep or refreshing. Without hormone support, you will have a shorter life span. You will also have a greater chance of developing vaginal and urinary infections, deeper skin creases, and hair loss. You will still have a one in nine chance of developing breast cancer.

It is really all about balance and common sense.

1

Understanding Health and Hormones

Let's face it, we all take our health for granted, yet without good health we have nothing. We run through our busy, overachieving lives at top speed and are amazed when somewhere in our late thirties or forties suddenly we notice that despite being bone tired, we just can't sleep and we don't have the same enthusiasm for the people we love. We notice other things, such as joints that don't withstand step classes, an extra roll of fat framing our belly button, or simply a dampening of our youthful glow. In our thirties, we women cope quite well, thank you very much. Pregnancy, menstrual cramps, monthly surges, and plunging hormones—we cope. How? We have youth. We are rich in hormones to buoy us up. But we take our hormones for granted, and when we hit our forties (and in some cases even our thirties) things start to change. Depending on how good our genetics, lifestyle, and environment are, our changes can be graceful or extreme. If our environment is neglected and toxic, watch out, our perimenopause or menopausal years will be tumultuous, sort of like a sudden global warming.

13

We women are hormonally diverse creatures. Most women in their forties don't think that they are candidates for using hormones. Sure, thirty- or forty-something women are thinking about exercise and vitamins, but not hormones. And who can blame them? Hormones have taken on a scary aura in the press. Athletes are disgraced for using them. We are frightened by reports of cancer and strokes. But I am not talking about athlete-level megadoses of hormones here. I am talking about learning what is right for you to maintain balance and feel great. This book is about learning what too little hormone feels like, and understanding why our levels are low and how we can restore hormones safely to normal levels.

When to Start Thinking about Supporting Your Hormones

You should start to think about supporting your hormones when you start noticing that you just aren't feeling as good as you used to. You don't want to wait until your bones are thinning and you've lost your hair, thinned your skin, and deepened your creases. You certainly don't want to wait until your arteries are damaged and your memory is failing. The fourth and fifth decades are the ideal time to start looking at your hormones. Why? Because we are biologically programmed to begin to die within ten years after childbearing ceases by a natural slow decline in our hormone levels.

From an evolutionary point of view, there is no great reason for us to stick around beyond childbirth. Evolution isn't influenced by 401Ks or the joys of grandchildren. Evolution is very shortsighted when it comes to aging. I am often asked, "Isn't supporting hormones unnatural? Weren't we supposed to just stop producing them and age gracefully, naturally?" Well, yes, it is true that we are meant to gradually produce fewer hormones as we age; and, yes, it is part of the aging process. But exciting things are happening. Life expectancy is increasing. The median life expectancy has now risen to 77.6 years, compared with 58 years in 1930.

Medical advances such as antibiotics, vaccinations, clot-dissolving medications, and "unnatural" techniques such as coronary bypass grafting have pushed back the grim reaper every year since 1950. That is both good news and bad news. If you look at the quality of life of most eighty-year-olds and beyond, it is not great. Many of us are not aging gracefully, and many of us are reaching our older age more burned out than our unliberated mothers, who didn't have the luxuries of career, family, and technology running them ragged. So we may live longer, but we have a good chance of suffering from Parkinson's, dementia, bone loss, or depression, not to mention bad skin and lots of body aches. It is estimated that in twenty years there will be more than one million people living longer than one hundred years. But who wants to get there hormonally deprived, with a feeble mind, heart, and bones, and with a sagging chin and no hair on your head?

This is why I, an overachieving, overscheduled fellow baby boomer and menopausal woman, spend my days lecturing women about hormones and vitamins and balance—so that our eighties and beyond can be healthier and more fun.

Hormonal decline is typically a slow, gradual decline in all of our hormones for both women and men. We refer to this phase of life as perimenopause in women and andropause in men. These are milestones leading to our older age. I like to think of these phases as the adolescence of old age. Do you recall how tough adolescence was? Well, in perimenopause it is happening all over again, only in reverse. Although hormonal decline is inevitable, it is not irreversible and it needn't be uncomfortable. We can ease it and even delay it.

How hormones decline is individualized. It may be quite noticeable in some but not in others. Most women feel their first symptoms during their forties, when adrenal and sex hormones begin to fall; but some women experience symptoms earlier, as a result of a stressful life event such as illness, divorce, or the death of a loved one. Infertility treatments can actually accelerate hormonal decline, as many protocols attempt to suppress a woman's natural hormonal cycle. This doesn't mean you shouldn't undergo fertility treatments—just be aware that your periods might wane or you might experience hot flashes afterward. Infertility is hard enough. Coupled with menopause, it can feel unbearable.

Bette Davis sure got it right when she said "Getting old ain't for sissies." It is estimated that during both perimenopause and menopause,

80 percent of all women suffer significant life-altering symptoms such as fatigue, depression, low sex drive, hot flashes, vaginal dryness, recurrent urinary or vaginal infections, insomnia, and more. As we get older, many things change. Our sleep is lighter, as our minds seem more prone to worry and upset. Our moods are often more erratic. Our bodies feel as if they are growing out of control, as if someone gave us too much fertilizer; our hips grow an extra handle; and for many women breasts ache and swell an extra bra size, only to wither and sag a year or two later. Nights can be long and lonely in perimenopause and menopause, and days can feel equally challenging. Sleep can become a second job. It is unreliable and erratic. Some nights it is impossible to fall asleep, and when at last a dream arises we are suddenly wide awake. Problems seem bigger and more difficult to untangle in the night, and hot flashes and body aches are usually worse then, too.

Women tolerate less as they age. Thelma and Louise sum up perimenopause. Would they have been different on hormones? Well, they definitely would have driven a Thunderbird and had great sex with Brad Pitt, but there probably would have been less killing. In your thirties, you may be willing to make do with a stale marriage or unfulfilling job, but by the time you hit your late forties most women are planning a change: new friends, new job, new clothes. Why do you think they call it "The Change"? You don't have the same tolerance at fifty that you may have had at thirty. Then you were busy building your empire, big or small, and you needed feedback and a pat on the back. As menopause approaches, with the empire built (and most likely up for sale), you just don't want to hear what anyone has to say about it.

Years ago there were ways to deal with women undergoing The Change—we were termed "hysterics" and were "asylumnized" or sent to the country for a rest. Nowadays we are put on Prozac or Celexa and given Ativan.

Well, it's a new millennium and a turning point for women's heath. We baby boomers who legalized abortion, revolutionized birth control, and pushed for double careers have learned a thing or two. With the good and bad of our endeavors, we are now in the midst of menopause. It is time to take charge of our health and perhaps even make things easier for our daughters, when their time comes.

Hormone Support Therapy

Hormone replacement therapy, or HRT, which was the main form of hormone therapy in the past, never made sense to me. Why replace hormones when you can support them naturally? Natural hormones (or bioidentical hormones) are identical to those found in nature. They look and act exactly the same as hormones that are made naturally in our bodies. They are not something new or foreign working in your body. Your own hormones are not replaced by synthetic, stronger-acting hormones. Women's hormones should certainly not be replaced by horse hormones.

I talk to my patients about hormone support therapy, or HST. Instead of replacing hormones, I recommend supporting them. Our adrenal glands were meant to produce our own sex hormones as we age. Anytime I put a woman on hormones, I support her adrenal hormones as well. Because the adrenals work in sync with the thyroid glands, it is important to make sure that both the thyroid and adrenal glands are working optimally. This will help you not only feel and look better, but you will have more energy and handle stress without falling apart. This is the basis for the natural hormone makeover. Support hormones naturally, and then "support the supports" with vitamins, minerals, and amino acids that control and regulate hormones. The final part of this hormone makeover is meant to ensure that your diet and lifestyle are helping you to safely metabolize, or process, your hormones, which can counteract the genetic and environmental risks of cancer and heart disease.

Hormone Fears

We live in a confusing time. It is hard to know whom and what to believe. Even the number of planets is controversial. In 1930 Pluto was considered a planet, but now it has been demoted to "probably a moon of Neptune." In 1982 all menopausal women were told to take Prempro or risk insanity and heart problems, but now if you take it you will be doomed to breast cancer and stroke. Recommendations seem to be changing every day. Once hormones were in, then they were out, and now they may actually be coming back in again, for a limited time— sort of like clunky shoes and leggings.

Most people refuse to take hormones out of fear of cancer or some other horrible disease. But let's take a look at hormones with some common sense. If estrogen and progesterone caused breast cancer, then pregnant women, adolescents, and young adults would have the very highest breast cancer rates because their bodies have the highest levels of these hormones. To the contrary, cancer rates increase with age, when our estrogen and progesterone levels are at their all-time low.

The one study that fomented a great deal of fear about breast cancer and heart disease from hormone use was the WHI study, published in 2002. (This study and others are discussed in more detail in chapters 3 and 9.)

What did the WHI study actually prove? Well, first you have to understand studies in general. For example, a recent study was published (by a man) supposedly proving that men are smarter than women. This study was conducted because it was observed that the man's brain weighs 100 grams more than a woman's, so it seemed obvious that men should have more brainpower. To prove this hypothesis, the researcher looked at college entrance SAT scores for men and women and found that men surpassed women in both verbal and mathematics (although the verbal scores were close). This news made headlines and got top billing on the morning talk shows. But there are many explanations. First of all, more women attend college than men. If you count men not in college—who didn't take SAT tests—the male scores will actually fall far lower, "proving" that women are in fact smarter. Studies often are like this. You need to compare apples with apples.

Many hormone studies are not unlike the study done to prove that men are smarter than women. The WHI study, for example, included women over many age ranges. But if you look only at the women aged fifty to fifty-nine years of age in the study, you find no increased risk of breast cancer and less heart disease in women on estrogen compared with women not taking hormones.

The fact remains that women who have high hormone levels (which occurs during pregnancy and adolescence) have little risk of developing cancer or heart disease. Common sense, then, would lead to the prediction that hormones protect against cancer, right? Well, this is indeed the case, despite the reports to the contrary. Why the discrepancy? It is because the most widely publicized hormone studies yielding negative results used synthetic hormones given by mouth to women who were more than ten years after menopause, many of whom already had signs of heart disease. These studies did not look at hormones that occur naturally inside a woman at the time when she needs them most—during perimenopause and immediately following menopause, before the effects of low hormones affect her cells.

Synthetic hormones cannot and should not be equated with the hormones naturally produced and metabolized in your own body. Synthetic progesterone (Provera or medroxyprogesterone) used in the now infamous WHI study has been shown for years to be carcinogenic (both to the breast and the ovaries) and to have other properties that can lead to excess clotting and heart problems. Synthetic progesterone has been shown to negate most positive estrogen effects on the heart, lipids, and blood vessels. It was synthetic progesterone that was found to correlate with an increase in both heart disease and breast cancer (the estrogen-only part of the study had less of both of these), yet somehow estrogen and all women's sex hormones got lumped together and blamed for the bad effects of synthetic progesterone. Hormones have been misrepresented, and women are now more confused and more uncomfortable than ever.

It is true that hormones are potent; used improperly, they can have ill effects. But in addition to considering the type of hormone used, you have to factor in how the hormones are taken, as well as environment, diet, and lifestyle. Estrogen taken by mouth (as was the case in the WHI study) increases blood clotting problems; estrogen taken through the skin (transdermally) does not increase clotting risks. All hormones are metabolized, or broken down, in our cells (particularly our breast and liver cells), and our hormone breakdown products (metabolites) leave our body through our stool and urine. How well we break down and excrete our hormones, particularly estrogen (which is the most difficult hormone to metabolize), is affected by our diet, bowels, environment, and genetics. If you are overweight or have a family history of poor estrogen metabolism, if your system is overwhelmed by clearing toxins, drugs, caffeine, or alcohol, or if your bowels are not moving regularly, there are bound to be problems. You have to consider the individual. If you have a family history of breast cancer or ovarian cancer, it doesn't mean that you can't take hormones, but it does mean that you need to pay attention to how the hormones work inside you. Breast cancer is largely an environmental illness due to poor environmental and lifestyle exposures that predispose to dangerous estrogen metabolites.

Hormones should be used in a balanced and monitored way. Hormones and their breakdown products should be measured before and during hormone use so that you can follow how the hormones are working inside your body. We all vary in size, build, genetics, diet, habits, environment, and metabolism; bowels and livers work better in some compared with others. Our hormone needs change as we age, gain or lose weight, deal with stress, or eat differently. For these reasons, your hormone dose should and will vary as you age and change. The hormone support for a forty-year-old woman who is still cycling (menstruating) will be different than for a fifty-five-year-old post-menopausal woman. It is important to understand how too much or too little of each hormone feels to be able to know when to increase or begin to taper off any hormone support you are using. This is why using a compounding pharmacist to give you hormone creams or lotions makes so much sense. Compounded hormone doses are individualized and allow you to change the dose as you need to, based on how you feel.

The Natural Hormone Makeover outlines ten steps to improve your health using natural hormones safely. Take a hard look at yourself to decide if your sleep, energy, and sense of well-being are as good as they could be, as good as you want them to be. Don't wait until you are having physical problems from hormone decline. Many women suffer from uterine fibroids with blood loss and hysterectomies, breast cysts, or even breast cancer due to poor hormone metabolism and progesterone deficiency. Bone loss, insomnia, depression, low sex drive, and fatigue, not to mention dry, aging skin and hair, are also the result of hormone loss. These problems can be halted or prevented with a sensible natural hormone program. Don't be frightened by studies that seem to change with the tides and manipulate statistics. Use common sense and see how you feel; this matters more than any study. It is up to you to take control of your own body, using hard facts. If we believe that natural hormones, used properly, cause cancer, we may as well believe that men are smarter than women. So forget all the studies you've read about (I promise to address them, though). The most important study is the study of your own unique body.

The Ten-Step Hormone Makeover

The goal is to get you to better understand how your body works so that you can look and feel better. Your body declines for many reasons, but hormonal decline is one of the main reasons that you age. By supporting your hormones safely and restoring normal levels, you can have more energy and enthusiasm, better-looking skin, stronger muscles, bones, and hair, and even better sex. Here are the ten basic steps to your hormone makeover:

1. **Know your symptoms.** You may think you are just fine, but if you are reading this book then you may be wondering how much better you could feel. Sometimes we think symptoms are normal, part of getting older. For example, you may be tired every day at 4 p.m. and think, "Oh well, that's life." Or you may wake every night at 3 a.m. and think, "That's what happens when you get older." It may not have dawned on you that these are in fact symptoms of weak adrenals or low thyroid hormones.

Symptoms are signs that things are out of balance. Painful, swollen breasts a week or two before your period aren't just part of being a woman. They are a sign that your progesterone is too low or your estrogen breakdown is not great. Pain and swelling in your breasts indicate inflammation and fluid retention. Insomnia that gets worse before your period is another sign of progesterone deficiency. We all know that hot flashes are a sign of low estrogen, but most women don't realize that low estrogen commonly causes migraines, hair loss, facial hair, and recurring urinary tract infections. How well you age depends a lot on how well your hormones are balanced. Recognize your symptoms and learn why you are having them in order to achieve balance.

Our bodies, particularly our hormones, bear the brunt of our lifestyle choices. We are for the most part overstimulated and overworked. We live in a world that is high in stress, and we eat foods that are high in fat and processed in such a way that removes many of the beneficial vitamins, fiber, and antioxidants. Our sleep is often disturbed or just plain too short. Symptoms hold the key to knowing which hormones are out of whack. By heeding and addressing our symptoms, we can feel and look much better. Being overweight, wrinkled, tired, and depressed is not normal. If you can't sleep, don't just take a sleeping pill and mask the underlying cause—check your hormone levels. Support what's low and look at your lifestyle to see what you can do to improve your hormones. Medications have their place, but the danger is that symptoms can be masked. Left untreated, imbalances will not be addressed, and over time new symptoms will arise or old symptoms will recur.

2. **Partner with a doctor and/or a compounding pharmacist.** Fortunately, more and more drug companies are marketing natural versions of estrogen, progesterone, and testosterone. But not all doctors are trained in using natural hormones. If you don't know whom to contact, try asking a compounding pharmacy what doctors are using natural hormones. Compounding pharmacies can be found in every state. By going online at IACP (International Academy of Compounding Pharmacies) you can readily find a compounding pharmacist near you. (Recommended pharmacies

are listed at the end of chapter 7.) Even if a compounding pharmacy is not near you, one can mail-order hormones and either work with your doctor or refer you to a nearby physician. Specialty labs (listed in chapter 6) that measure hormone levels are also great sources for finding a doctor in your area.

3. **Measure your hormone levels and do baseline tests.** Although your symptoms can help determine if hormones are out of balance, you need to measure hormone levels to determine precisely which hormones are responsible. The adrenal gland produces many hormones, and typically more than one will be low. Sometimes the problem can be too much of a hormone. For example, your cortisol may be low or normal in the morning but very high at night, making it impossible to fall or stay asleep. For that matter, when some hormones are low, others may rise to compensate, as so often happens with thyroid and adrenal hormones. That is why lab testing must be done for you, a unique individual, with your own symptoms in mind.

   What's too high or too low? What's normal? Many physicians are trained to treat only those hormones that are below normal ranges. But normal ranges are not always clear and may not be appropriate for your particular age or size. Often the normal ranges are just too broad. Surely the normal hormone level for a two-hundred-pound, fifty-year-old woman is not going to be the same as normal for an eighty-five-pound eighty-year-old. Yet the same values are often given for all adult women regardless of age, size, or metabolism.

   Consider also that normal is not a precise amount but a range from low-normal to high-normal. Why wait for a hormone to actually fall below normal levels and adversely affect how your cells function? It is best to support hormones that are below midrange before they become deficient. Hormone levels can be measured in your blood, saliva, or urine. Which test you use will depend upon your insurance coverage and what your doctor recommends.

   Typically before starting hormone support for my patients, I measure all adrenal and thyroid hormones as well as the minerals that affect hormone function (that is, iron, calcium, and magnesium). These are not exotic or unusual tests. You don't necessarily need to measure estrogen or progesterone right off the bat if you are no longer cycling, because you know and expect that these will be low. Estrogen and progesterone should be measured, however, if you are cycling or have stopped cycling unexpectedly. Melatonin, growth hormone, and nighttime cortisol should be checked if you are having insomnia that has not responded to simply supporting your sex hormones.

Baseline tests such as mammograms, bone density scans, and ultrasounds are also important. I always recommend that women have a mammogram and bone density scan within a year of starting hormone support. A woman who is menopausal and not on hormone support will typically lose 3 percent of her bone mass each year. For this reason, I like to see where the bones are starting from to help advise about continuing therapies in the coming years. If you have bone loss, and in spite of strength training, calcium, vitamins D and K, bone minerals, and estrogen and progesterone, your bone density doesn't improve after around a full year of sex hormone support, you may want to expand your hormone support to include growth hormone. You might also consider digestive causes (insufficient fat or protein absorption). If you have a history of uterine fibroids, I recommend getting a pelvic ultrasound to see if hormone use has caused any further growth of fibroids—which shouldn't happen if your support is well balanced.

4. **Start by supporting sex hormones.** Because the sex hormones (estrogen and progesterone in women) affect nearly every major symptom, including sleep, energy, mood, sex drive, and general sense of well-being, it makes sense to support these first. How will you know if your sex hormones are balanced? You'll know because your menstrual or menopausal symptoms will be better. You should notice that your sex drive has increased, and that you have little or no PMS. Hot flashes should stop, and you should feel a sense of well-being. Your sleep should be deeper, and intercourse should be comfortable. Your energy should be much better, and even your hair should feel stronger. Over time your skin will wrinkle less, particularly around your mouth and eyes. Your skin, your vagina, your eyes, and even your joints should become

more lubricated, and you will begin to look younger. Sex hormones won't reverse aging that has already taken place, but they will lessen aging effects in the future.

5. **Support adrenal and thyroid hormones.** These hormones support and help to regulate sex hormones. You can pretty much assume that you will need some adrenal support if your sex hormones are out of whack, because the adrenals are supposed to support your sex hormones as you age. Treating adrenal and thyroid imbalances together is often the fine-tuning part of the makeover. Although most women feel better on sex hormone support alone, most really start to feel great once their thyroid and adrenal glands are working optimally. Their energy, mood, anxiety, allergies, and even muscle aches improve.

   There are many adrenal hormones, such as DHEA, cortisol, pregnenolone, aldosterone, and epinephrine, all of which affect our energy, sleep, and mood. Usually more than one is needed for various periods of time. Your thyroid gland works closely with your adrenal gland. If your thyroid function is low, adrenal hormones, particularly cortisol and sometimes aldosterone, may rise to compensate. Over time this can lead to high blood pressure and a lowered adrenal reserve. This explains why many women initially feel very good on thyroid hormones, with improved morning energy, but over a matter of weeks start to feel tired once again, particularly late in the day. Similarly, if the adrenal hormones are low, the thyroid may respond by producing excess hormones, leading to a sense of anxiety and heart palpitations.

6. **Measure melatonin and growth hormone levels.** These two hormones are more difficult to measure, and not all doctors agree about the best way to measure them, but these hormones should be considered if your sleep is still not deep, consistent, and refreshing. Melatonin improves sleep and also reduces the signs of aging on the face. In addition, it can lessen your feelings of anxiety. Growth hormone also helps to reduce anxiety, and it too deepens sleep and prevents many aging effects on the face, such as a dwindling upper lip, shrinking jawline, and deepening skin creases. In addition, growth hormone enhances sex drive, helps redistribute weight, restores bone density, and improves muscle and bone strength.

7. **Support the supports with vitamins, herbs, minerals, and amino acids, as well as a healthy diet and lifestyle.** Surprisingly, adrenal, thyroid, and sex hormones are made from cholesterol and amino acids and require specific vitamins, minerals, essential fatty acids, and protein for optimal function. By supporting the supports, you may eventually be able to lower or even withdraw hormone support altogether. It is not surprising that we are seeing epidemic hormone deficiencies in a society preoccupied with lipid-lowering drugs, low-fat diets, and highly processed, artificially fortified fast foods. Diet and lifestyle play a significant role in our hormone levels, and may be why levels became low in the first place.

8. **Monitor your hormone metabolism.** To make sure that hormone support is safe, hormone metabolites should be measured annually for some hormones, particularly estrogen and DHEA, to ensure that your hormones are breaking down safely inside you. Hormone metabolism has only recently begun to be understood. Consequently, such monitoring is not currently routine, but it should be. It can help to lessen adverse side effects from hormones and may even be lifesaving. Most hormones are activated and/or broken down in the liver. From the liver, hormones are passed into the digestive tract in the bile to be excreted. It makes sense, then, that if your bowels are sluggish or if your liver is busy breaking down pesticides, pollutants, toxins, caffeine, alcohol, cigarette smoke, or other drugs, things can go wrong. Harmful metabolites place you at greater risk for hormone-related cancers. Genetics play a big role here. How you break down hormones is handed down in your genes. Fortunately, genetic tendencies can be helped with the right dietary choices and supplements. Diet, properly used supplements, and changes in your environment can help ensure that hormones will act safely inside your body.

9. **Taper off support (or not).** With proper nutritional, supplemental, and lifestyle supports, your body will be brought back into balance. Your body may produce more of its own hormones. If you have excess hormones, you will develop symptoms such as breast tenderness, feeling too energetic or anxious, or a return of

insomnia. This is not a bad thing, but it can be confusing. If your levels become too high while on support, this is a sign that your body's own hormone levels have improved and you can begin to taper off or change your support to a lower dose of hormones or a less strong herbal or vitamin support.

10. **Maintain your health as you age.** People are confused about how and when to have tests to monitor hormones. Tests such as mammograms, Pap smears, bone density scans, and measuring markers of aging such as fasting insulin levels, SHBG (sex-hormone-binding globulin), and even antioxidants can be done, but when and how often? Despite published guidelines, monitoring should be individualized depending on what hormonal support you need, your risk factors, and your genetics. If your bone density is low, don't wait five years to recheck it; recheck it in one year to make sure that your natural hormone support is working to restore bone. Pap smears may not need to be done annually if "high-risk" HPV (human papilloma virus) cultures taken during your Pap smear are normal (ask your doctor to check). Some tests, such as mammograms and metabolite measuring, should be done each year to ensure a safe makeover experience.

As you can see, understanding what hormones do and what it feels like when hormones are not in balance is important to feel your best and to slow down the natural aging process. I hope that this will be the beginning of a better understanding of just who you are and why you feel the way you do.

Hormone Safety and Metabolism

Hormones have been around since women first walked this Earth. They have not changed, but how we view them has varied widely. Women's hormones have become almost mythical, taking on a life of their own in our daily media, sometimes bestowed with great powers and at other times degraded and feared. The myriad of hormone studies are overwhelming and confusing, and lately women don't know what to do or whom to trust. I have studied ancient therapies, worked with cutting-edge technologies, and lived through perimenopause myself. I have reviewed a multitude of studies, and in this chapter I will try to demystify hormones for you by looking at several of these studies with calm and common sense.

I recommend that all women support their hormones if they have symptoms during perimenopause and continue that support for at least the first ten years of menopause, and possibly beyond. Timing, the type of hormone used, and how hormones are broken down inside your body determine many of their risks. Hormone breakdown, or metabolism, is like a waste treatment facility located primarily in your liver. How well your toxic waste is handled depends on your genetics, diet, and environment. Chinese medicine recognized centuries ago that proper diet and a balanced lifestyle could improve poor ancestral, or inherited, tendencies and alleviate hormonal symptoms. In addition to shedding light on some of the large hormone studies, this chapter will explain hormone metabolism, why hormones should be used, and how they can be used safely. I hope you will come to understand why the Chinese say, "A happy liver makes for a happy woman."

The Big, Bad Studies: Not the Whole Story

Many large-scale studies have looked at the safety of women's sex hormones. Unfortunately, the largest studies in this country have primarily examined the safety and benefits of synthetic hormones taken orally. Such studies do not tell the whole story because the hormones used were not the same as the hormones naturally found inside you, a living, breathing actual woman. Before you take the results of such studies to heart, understand four important points: (1) The type of estrogen used in most of these studies was horse estrogen. (2) The hormones were given by mouth, not via the skin (transdermally). (3) The progesterone used was a synthetic form, usually medroxyprogesterone, which is not the same as a woman's own natural progesterone. (4) The timing for hormone support is important—it must be given before diseases such as heart disease and detrimental brain effects occur. Let me address these points and then take a look at the studies.

First, guess what? Horses are different from women. Horse estrogen fuels the eleven-month pregnancy of a twelve-hundred-pound mare, as she gains about two hundred pounds. It is one heck of a lot stronger than a woman's own estrogen. And it should come as no surprise that horse estrogen does not metabolize normally in women. It is broken down in a woman's body into over forty estrogen-like metabolites, many of which are harmful and have been linked to breast cancer (not unlike DES, diethylstilbestrol, another horse estrogen knockoff, which was banned in 1971 after it was linked to an increase in cancer in the women using it and in the offspring of such women who were exposed to it in utero).

Second, horse hormones (and women's hormones, too) are not a food source. They are not intended to be eaten (taken orally). Hormones are produced in glands and secreted directly into the bloodstream. When hormones are eaten, they travel directly to the liver for processing. This has many bad consequences. Because the liver is where clotting proteins develop, hormones given orally increase blood clotting. This doesn't happen when hormones are given transdermally, through the skin. Hormones taken through the skin are gradually absorbed into the bloodstream, much the way hormones produced naturally in your glands would be. High hormone levels do not overwhelm your liver, and excess clotting does not occur. Many studies have consistently shown that transdermal estrogen does not significantly increase blood clotting the way oral estrogen does. High levels of hormones in the liver also cause the body to make large amounts of binding proteins that can lower your thyroid, estrogen, and testosterone, defeating their very purpose.

Third, synthetic progesterone is carcinogenic and has been linked to breast and ovarian cancer; your natural progesterone is not cancer-causing. Synthetic progesterone is vastly different from your own natural progesterone, produced by your ovaries to counteract the stimulating effect that estrogen has on your cells—particularly on the cells lining your uterus and inside your breasts. Natural progesterone is referred to as the pregnancy hormone, which is when it is particularly important for balancing the very high levels of estrogen that are circulating (discussed more fully in chapter 8).

Natural progesterone has never been shown to be carcinogenic. If it were, pregnant women, who have the highest levels of all, would be getting cancer left and right, but they do not. To the contrary, numerous studies have shown that natural progesterone has protective effects against cancer, and that women who lack progesterone during perimenopause have an increased risk of breast cancer. Natural progesterone prevents blood clotting and the narrowing of blood vessels, which can be caused by high levels of estrogen. In addition, natural progesterone reduces bad lipids and improves good lipids, but synthetic progestins don't. Synthetic progesterone behaves like an "antiprogesterone." Odd as this may seem, women taking synthetic progesterones, known as progestins, look and feel like women who have too little progesterone. They complain of tender, swollen breasts, fluid retention, headaches, and bloating.

Finally, the timing of hormones is important. Deaths from heart disease double between the ages of forty-five and fifty-five, and again from fifty-five to sixty-five, and then increase twelvefold from age seventy-five to eighty-four. Remember, we human beings are programmed to begin to die once our childbearing years are over. Consequently, the inevitable gradual hormonal decline in our forties and fifties leads to an acceleration of vessel disease, increasing our risk of heart disease, hypertension, stroke, and dementia. Most women will develop heart disease by age sixty, and once it starts, hormones cannot reverse it. Natural progesterone has been shown experimentally to reduce brain degeneration and even Parkinson's disease. You need to take hormones to prevent the diseases of aging before they begin. You need hormones most during perimenopause and for the first ten years of menopause.

Why You Are Scared

All of this doesn't mean you can ignore the studies. They have something to tell us if we dig beneath the media hype and horror. Here is what you need to know about some of the largest, most widely publicized hormone studies:

The Nurses' Health Study (NHS), funded by the National Institutes of Health (NIH), has two parts and is still ongoing. The first part, started in 1976, followed 122,000 nurses aged thirty to fifty-five. The second, started in 1989, followed 116,000 nurses aged twenty-five to forty-two. These are the longest studies on women's health ever done, and they are important because they began with women in their thirties, forties and fifties who took synthetic hormones for birth control or symptoms of perimenopause or menopause. Hormones were started before these women reached the high-risk years for heart disease, stroke, and dementia, which could skew the results. There have been over 250 papers reporting on observations from these two groups. Here are some of the highlights:

- Women had a greater likelihood of living longer if they used hormones. Mortality rates were 37 percent lower in women who used hormones. After ten years of hormone use, this mortality rate was 20 percent lower.

- In the first ten years of hormone use, women who developed breast cancer had a lower death rate than women who developed breast cancer without using hormones.
- There were 40 to 50 percent fewer heart attacks in menopausal women who used estrogen. Heart disease reduction continued up to seventy-one years of age.
- Synthetic hormones increased breast cancer risk by 33 percent.
- Consuming one to three drinks of alcohol increased the incidence of breast cancer by 30 percent. This increases further if consuming more than three drinks per day.
- Calcium supplements taken alone, without hormones, did not reduce bone fractures.

The Heart/Progestin Replacement Study (HERS), published in 1998, was funded by Wyeth-Ayerst laboratories, the makers of Prempro (a combination of Premarin, synthetic horse estrogen, and Provera, synthetic medroxyprogesterone). This study followed 2,763 post-menopausal women with an average age of sixty-seven. In this age group, despite small improvements in good cholesterol and some lowering of bad cholesterol, Prempro failed to reduce heart disease, compared with women not taking any hormones. Additional bad news was an increase in blood clots in the veins of the legs and the lungs and a small increase in stroke. So kiss your Prempro good-bye.

The Million Women Study recruited 1,084,110 women living in the United Kingdom between 1996 and 2001. This was actually not a controlled clinical study, but a survey of women's hormone use and outcome regarding breast cancer. The women taking hormones were using either oral contraceptives, Prempro, Premarin alone, or Tibilone (a synthetic drug that mimics both estrogen and progesterone). More than 50 percent of the women were older than fifty-six. This survey showed an increase in breast cancer in women using synthetic hormones. Again, more bad news about synthetic hormones and breast cancer.

The Women's Health Initiative study, published in 2002, was funded by the U.S. government to study two different hormone therapies and their effects on heart disease and breast cancer. This study fueled most of the bad press on hormones and resulted in over 7 million women of all ages suddenly quitting hormones completely.

The WHI study was unique because it followed women who didn't have symptoms of menopause (so that the dropout rate would be low). But using women who had few or no symptoms skewed the study because women without menopausal symptoms tended to be older. Of the 160,000 women studied, the average age was sixty-seven, and 21 percent of the women were well over seventy years old. Because of their older age, many of these women already had heart disease risk factors (abnormal blood lipids, hypertension), and some women had a history of heart disease. Some women in the WHI study were given Prempro, other women (who had had hysterectomies) were given Premarin alone, and the remainder were given placebos without any hormone content. The Prempro arm of the study was halted three years early (after only five years) because of a 26 percent increase in breast cancers and a 29 percent increase in heart attacks. This sounds like a lot, but the group without hormones also had an increase. It actually works out to 8 more breast cancers and 7 more heart attacks for every 10,000 women using hormones. Other findings were a 50 percent increase in blood clots (18 more cases) and a 41 percent increase in stroke (8 more cases). The good news was that there were fewer bone fractures and less colon cancer, and despite the increases in cancer and clots, the mortality rate was actually lower in the Prempro group compared with the placebo group.

The WHI study was meant to provide information about the use of hormones in menopause, but instead it generated more heat than light. Unfortunately, after the Prempro arm of the study was ended prematurely, mass hysteria ensued. Millions of women went off all hormone replacement. Two years after the first reports, the Premarin-only group reports were released to little fanfare despite some very encouraging results (including less heart disease in women using estrogen alone, particularly women aged fifty to fifty-nine). Many hormone-positive critiques and reevaluations of the studies have been published. Unfortunately, few of these critiques have made their way to the people who most need them: menopausal women, particularly those who are within ten years of postmenopause, who really should be taking natural hormones.

Despite the criticisms and debate, the good news about hormones was overshadowed by the bad; and subsequent positive studies of other parts of the WHI study received little attention.

To summarize, here is what these large studies show:

- The Nurses' Health Study tells us that women live longer if they use hormones (even synthetics) when compared with women not using hormones. As a woman ages, her risk of heart disease increases, and using hormones early on, before age sixty, lowers heart disease risk and lowers mortality despite a slightly higher risk of developing breast cancer if using synthetic hormones. These studies also found that drinking alcohol significantly increases the risk of breast cancer.
- The HERS study tells us that when using oral, synthetic horse estrogen and synthetic progesterone over the age of sixty, there is no reduction in heart disease but there is an increased risk of blood clots and stroke. It also shows that women with a history of heart attack have an increased risk of heart disease during the first year of hormone treatment.
- The Million Women Study tells us that using synthetic hormones increases the risk of breast cancer.
- Subsequent evaluations of the WHI data demonstrate that even synthetic estrogen reduced heart disease in women if given in the first ten years of menopause. In addition, in all ages it reduces bone fractures, colon cancer, and mortality rates. The bad news from the WHI is that use of medroxyprogesterone (Provera) is associated with an increase in breast cancer and heart disease. In all ages, oral synthetic hormone use increases blood clots and stroke, and in women who start hormones more than ten years after menopause, hormone use does not reduce heart disease.

Timing of Hormones

The WHI study showed that the closer a woman was to menopause when she began using estrogen, the less likely she was to develop heart disease. This finding has provoked debate about the importance of when to start taking hormones, particularly for prevention of heart disease, dementia, and even Parkinson's disease. Timing has little to do with age and everything to do with falling hormone levels. For example, a fifty-four-year-old woman could have been menopausal for ten years or for two years, but what appears most critical is the amount of time she is menopausal. Brain cells, in particular, are susceptible to aging once hormone levels fall. Here are some snippets from recent studies that are interesting about the timing of hormones:

- In the WHI study, women who began using hormones within five years of menopause or hysterectomy had better memory scores when tested (all women tested were older than sixty).
- Women in the WHI study who began hormone replacement therapy (HRT) closer to menopause tended to have less heart disease than when HRT was started later. A substudy of these women's CAT scans showed less plaque (hardening of the arteries) in heart vessels when hormones were started early in menopause.
- A study of 1,889 women showed that if HRT was started within ten years of menopause and lasted for at least ten years, there was a significant reduction in dementia. But if women began their HRT ten years later, they had a greater risk of dementia. Other studies have also shown this.
- Experimentally, natural progesterone and natural estrogen protect dopamine pathways (important in Parkinson's). Studies have shown that the risk of Parkinson's disease increases in women with an early onset of menopause.
- Brain MRI studies have shown that the longer the duration of HRT, the better the brain tissues looked (less shrinkage of white and gray matter).

Breast Cancer Fears

Breast cancer is the most common reason that women refuse to use hormones, but what many women don't realize is that their body continues to make estrogen long after menopause. Deciding not to use any estrogen support does not protect a woman from breast cancer; many studies have clearly shown that. The older a woman is (and the lower her estradiol levels are), the more likely she is to get breast cancer. As the NHS study and other studies have shown, women not using estrogen who developed breast cancer fared worse (had a higher mortality rate, a more aggressive disease, and a poorer quality of life) than women who used hormone support. In a review of fifty-five studies about estrogen and breast cancer, forty-five studies concluded that estrogen use alone did not raise the risk of breast cancer; and there are now sixty published studies indicating that estrogen can be given safely to women with a history of breast cancer.

Natural progesterone can help prevent breast cancer. Studies have shown that the risk of developing breast cancer was decreased in women with naturally high levels of progesterone, and the risk of developing breast cancer was increased in women with low levels of midcycle progesterone.

You are probably thinking, How can that be? You have read headlines like: "Cancer Rates Plummet as Hormone Use Declines." But these rates were falling before the WHI study was released. And, yes, as the use of synthetic progesterone, Provera, and synthetic horse estrogen, Premarin, has fallen, cancer rates have further declined. But do not equate these synthetics with natural hormones, and disregard the numerous studies of estrogen used alone (without synthetic progestins) and breast cancer rates.

Bioidentical Hormones: Myth and Fact

So we know from the mega-studies, discussed above, many things about synthetic hormones, but what about natural, bioidentical hormones such as the hormones that are normally circulating in you? Are they safe?

Don't let anyone tell you that natural hormones are unproven, unsafe, uncontrolled, or unstudied. First of all, natural hormones have a great track record. Since time began, adolescents, who have the highest levels of sex hormones coursing through their bloodstream, have had the lowest rates of breast cancer, heart disease, and stroke. As a woman ages and her estrogen levels fall, these diseases and dementia increase steadily.

Bioidentical hormones have come under fire from many directions. Here are some of the common criticisms and my response:

- **Bioidentical hormones are derived from plants and have been described as natural, but they are not really natural if they are made in a lab.** Bioidentical hormones are natural, not because of where they come from, but because they look and behave just as our own natural hormones do. They will act at our cell receptors and break down in our cells (metabolize) exactly the same way as the estrogen and progesterone, naturally made inside our body, have always done. These hormones are derived from soy (or yam in some cases), but there is no human estrogen in soy. The phytoestrogens (plant compounds that look like estrogen) in soy must be chemically modified to become identical to our own natural estrogen.

- **Just because something is natural doesn't mean that it's safe.** That is correct. Many natural things are potentially toxic. Anything that you put in or on your body must be used wisely. Too many of one type of vitamin, too much of one type of hormone, even too much of certain foods can be toxic or harmful. This doesn't mean we shouldn't use natural supplements. We just need to use them wisely. For example, iron is natural, and doctors prescribe it routinely for anemia, but too much iron can damage your heart, liver, and other organs. We shouldn't shy away from a natural substance simply because it may not be safe if used incorrectly. Yes, too much estrogen can be dangerous. To make it safe it has to be used transdermally, in the proper dose, and balanced with progesterone.

- **Bioidentical hormones are not FDA-approved.** This is partly true and partly false. Bioidentical *compounded* hormones are not FDA-approved because they do not need to be. However, many bioidentical hormones are FDA-approved.

  Compounded hormone doses vary from individual to individual. They are individually tailored by physicians who spend years studying and training and whose qualifications and training are regulated by medical boards. It's not the FDA's job to oversee doctors. Compounded hormones prescribed by doctors are produced by compounding pharmacists who are regulated by pharmaceutical boards (see chapter 7). The FDA has approved certain standardized doses of bioidentical hormones that are not compounded for specific patients, such as bioidentical estradiol patches, testosterone gels, natural progesterone capsules, and vaginal creams. Such bioidentical hormones are FDA-approved and available to all women with a doctor's prescription.

  It is important to remember that FDA approval doesn't guarantee 100 percent safety. We have come to believe that the FDA has a rigorous system that ensures all products are safe and that an FDA seal of approval is like putting on a bulletproof vest when you take a medication. This is not the case. The FDA decides if a drug's benefits outweigh its risks. Once a drug is approved for marketing, the FDA watches to see if anything will go wrong. There are many FDA-approved drugs, that, over time, have caused serious problems. DES, Premarin, Thalidomide, and Vioxx, to name a few, were all FDA-approved but are now known to be associated with increased risks of cancer, blood clots, birth defects, and heart disease. FDA approval does not mean that no possible harm can come to you from using a medication.

● **There are no studies supporting the safety or efficacy of bioidentical hormones.** This is not true. Bioidentical hormones have been used by physicians in this country and worldwide for over twenty years. In the United States, bioidentical hormones are now available from drug companies, with hundreds of studies showing their efficacy in reducing heart disease risk factors, protecting women's uterine linings, and preventing waning bone densities. Studies using transdermal estrogen have not shown increases in blood clotting, as occurs with oral estrogen preparations (also discussed in chapter 9).

In Europe, women are commonly treated with transdermal estradiol gels and natural progesterone, and there are many well-conducted studies proving their efficacy and safety. In a French study published in 2002, more than three thousand women using transdermal bioidentical estradiol gel and natural progesterone were followed for nearly nine years. These women were shown to have an improved quality of life, less bone loss, and reduced heart disease risk without an increase in breast cancer or clotting. Another French study of 54,000 women using estrogen (oral and transdermal) and synthetic or natural progesterone showed that the risk of breast cancer was increased after only two years in the group using synthetic progesterone. No increase was seen when natural progesterone was used. This study was updated, and even after eight years of treatment, there was no increase in the natural progesterone group.

There are many other studies worldwide that support the use of natural hormones, with greater safety margins than synthetic hormones.

Hormone Metabolism

Bioidentical hormones are safe to use when their breakdown products, metabolites, are properly disposed of by your body. How well your body metabolizes, or breaks down, your estrogen largely determines your risk of breast cancer. Some estrogen metabolites are good and some are not so good. As you age, the type of estrogen that you produce shifts from a potent, sexy, moisturizing form (estradiol) to a weaker, less feminizing, possibly dangerous form (estrone). How well you metabolize your estrone largely determines how safe estrogen will be in you.

Metabolism of estrone is dependent on many things, including your genes, body weight, habits, environment, and diet. Alcohol, obesity, a family history of breast cancer, pesticides, synthetic progesterone, and environmental pollutants will raise your risk. A balanced lifestyle, normal body weight, regular exercise, and a diet rich in antioxidants and cruciferous vegetables can help to reduce your risk. How lifestyle affects your metabolism is the topic of chapter 4; this chapter will examine how your hormones are broken down.

Estrogen Metabolism

Women are usually amazed when I tell them that their body makes over a dozen forms of estrogen. Our understanding of the many forms of estrogen is still very new and ever-changing. It is certainly the most complicated of all hormones metabolically, which is why studies about her use can be so confusing. Estrogen metabolites are sometimes good and sometimes bad. As I mentioned, in our liver most estrogens convert into an estrone. A good estrone prevents your bones from crumbling and your vessels from becoming inflamed, thereby helping to ward off heart attacks and strokes. A good estrone will do you no harm and, in fact, will protect you from cancer, heart disease, bone loss, and memory loss. A bad estrone, on the other hand, can turn cells into cancer or make them grow into fibroids or cysts. It gives estrogen a bad reputation. So you need to produce lots of good estrones and not too many bad ones.

Meet the Estrones

Think of estrogen metabolites as in-laws. When you get married you think you are simply marrying one person, but you soon realize that with your spouse comes an entire package of in-laws, some great and some not so great. Like it or not, all estrones are part of the estrogen package. There are three important estrones to know about:

- **2-methoxyestrone (2-ME estrone)** is the beneficial form of estrogen responsible for most of the good things that we attribute to estrogen. I liken her to a fairy godmother bestowing strong bones, a clear mind, and a strong heart. The estrone 2-methoxyestrone (made from 2-OH estrone) prevents inflammation in the bones, brain, and heart vessels, thereby lowering your risk of dementia, osteoporosis, and heart disease. Whereas estrogen stimulates cells, particularly in the breast and uterus, 2-methoxyestrone (and 2-OH estrone) have been shown to limit cell growth. Women with a history of breast cancer or a family history of breast cancer typically have trouble making this estrone.

  In order for your body to make 2-methoxyestrone from 2-OH estrone, two things must happen: (1) Your diet must be rich in cruciferous vegetables, some soy products, and flax meal; and (2) your body must be able to methylate (discussed later), which requires vitamins B_6, B_{12}, and folic acid.

- **16-hydroxyestrone (16-OH estrone)** is poorly understood, but it may behave badly. I consider her a mysterious drama queen. This metabolite is short-lived in our circulation, where it readily converts into estriol. It has some good estrogen effects on the bones and possibly bad effects on other organs. Some studies report that she is capable of overstimulating the breast and the uterus and is possibly related to fibrocystic breast disease, ovarian cysts, fibroids, abnormal bleeding, and uterine hyperplasia. Some authorities claim that 16-OH estrone is carcinogenic, but its role in cancer is not clear. Although women with breast cancer (and their relatives) tend to have excess 16-OH estrone compared with 2-OH estrone, it is thought that the real problem is too little good 2-OH estrone, not necessarily the presence of 16-OH estrone. This is where cruciferous vegetables are so important. They contain a substance known as indole-3-carbinol, or I3C (discussed in chapter 4), which increases 2-OH estrone and limits 16-OH estrone. If you have a history of breast cancer or are genetically or otherwise predisposed to making too much 16-OH estrone (for example, a history of fibroids and cysts), you should supplement with I3C (400 mg/day).

- **4-hydoxyestrone (4-OH estrone)** is a potent estrogen metabolite. She is definitely the bully of all estrogens and the most feared, as she is considered to be a free radical generator capable of increasing your risk of dementia, heart disease, and breast cancer. Premarin and other horse estrogens (DES) cause high levels of 4-OH estrone to form. This estrone is not harmful by itself, but if it mixes with oxygen (becomes oxidized) it transforms into free radicals known as quinones. Quinones damage blood vessels and the DNA in cells. Studies have shown that even normal breast tissue, taken during surgery for breast cancer, contains higher than normal levels of 4-OH estrone and quinones.

Estrogen Metabolism

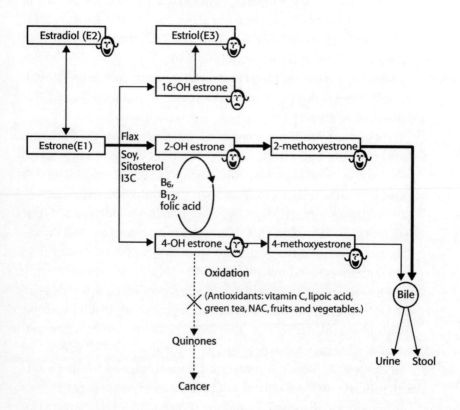

So you have learned a bit about the good and bad estrones. Now it's time to look at how you can improve your estrones, which are made in many of your cells, particularly your liver. Most estrogen metabolism takes place in the liver. It is amazing to me that Chinese medicine thousands of years ago appreciated liver metabolism and how to keep hormones safe. The Chinese understood that many women's health problems improved when the health of their liver improved. This may sound strange, but let me describe the liver as seen by Chinese medicine. I promise that it will shed light on many of your symptoms.

The Liver According to Chinese Medicine

The Chinese saying that a woman is as happy as her liver intrigued me when I first heard it. Based on all of the women that I had treated, I knew there were a lot of unhappy livers walking around, and I wanted to understand this from both the Chinese and Western perspectives.

In Chinese medicine, an organ is not just a body part. It is a pathway, called a meridian, and it is named for the organ that it nourishes. This idea is not far-fetched when you consider that our organs and limbs developed from specific regions when we were an embryo. For instance, a meridian in our arm is connected to our heart or lungs, which makes sense since our heart and lungs developed from the same place as our arms when we were an embryo. Our liver grew from the same embryologic region as our legs, hence the liver meridian begins in our foot.

According to Chinese medicine, our body's twelve meridians, or energetic pathways, nourish and regulate our organs, muscles, and nerves. The flow of energy through our meridians affects how we think and feel. I had a hard time conceptualizing meridians when I first studied Chinese medicine. I had done many surgeries and human dissections and studied all of the nerve and blood pathways, but I had never seen a meridian. Then one day in an art class, I had my "eureka" moment. When an artist paints, he must paint the "negative space," the seemingly empty area between objects. Meridians are the negative spaces, or the empty planes, between our organs, muscles, vessels, tendons, and lymph channels. This space is not truly empty; it is filled with fluids, rich in salts and minerals, with an electromagnetic charge and flow. The seemingly empty spaces of the body are constantly moving like a stream, flowing to nourish our organs and other body parts, as described by Chinese medicine. This electromagnetic charge, or movement through our meridians, is referred to by the Chinese as *qi* (pronounced "chee"), or vital force. Flow of our vital force through our meridians controls how well our organs, muscles, and lymph flow function. *Qi's* nature is to move. You don't want your *qi* to stagnate, or move poorly. Otherwise symptoms and disease result.

What does this have to do with hormone metabolism? The Chinese recognized centuries ago that the flow of *qi* through the liver meridian greatly affects women's health. Understand the liver meridian, and you will understand how to treat many of the problems that plague women.

The Liver Meridian

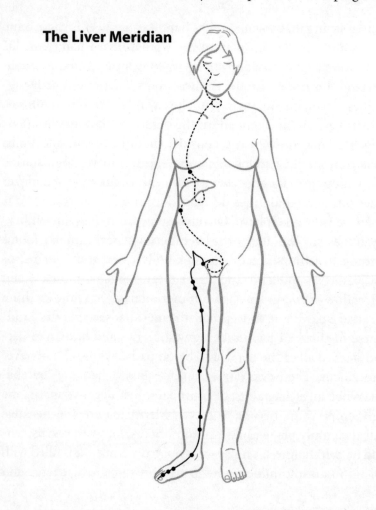

The liver meridian courses up the leg to the groin; then, after circling around the rectum and pelvis, it travels inwardly upward to wrap around the liver and gallbladder. It then proceeds up the chest, across the breasts and nipples, into the thyroid glands and eyes. Most women's health problems follow this same path. Women are particularly prone to problems in the pelvis (uterine fibroids and ovarian cysts), rectum (hemorrhoids), liver, gallbladder, breasts, and thyroid, and they often suffer from migraines coming from behind the eye.

The Chinese view of liver metabolism is poetic, with descriptions of flowing streambeds into clear tributaries. I use this analogy with patients to describe how their liver breaks down their hormones. If their rivers are clear and moving well, then their flow of hormones will be smooth and free-flowing. They will feel relaxed and calm, and if they are still cycling, their menstrual blood will flow evenly without pain, clots, or "floods." If there are stagnant streams with poor hormone metabolites, as may occur from excess caffeine, drugs, fatigue, pollutants, or stress, the river will flow poorly and some streams may overflow with water and debris, giving rise to tumultuous moods; swollen, tender breasts; headaches; and cramps from heavily flowing blood.

This liver congestion of which the Chinese speak so poetically can actually be seen when you look at lab reports of hormone metabolites. People who are taking excess hormones, living an unbalanced lifestyle, or taking too many prescription medications often have abnormally high or uneven hormone metabolites (measured in the urine), despite low hormone levels in the blood. Liver congestion, stagnant liver *qi*, is a syndrome well recognized in Chinese medicine, and it explains many symptoms commonly seen in women but often unexplained by Western medicine.

According to Chinese medicine, breast and thyroid disease are a problem with the liver. PMS symptoms are due to a stagnant, poor-moving liver *qi*. Other cultures recognize this as well. In fact, the dictionary defines "liverish" as being irritable or disagreeable. According to Chinese medicine, symptoms due to liver stagnation include irritability, depression, migraines, PMS, mood swings, atypical chest pains, abdominal bloating, hyperventilation syndrome, fibrocystic breast disease, headache, and irregular menstruation or menstrual cramps.

I think of metabolism as the biochemistry of the Chinese liver *qi*. If *qi* is flowing smoothly, then metabolism is working well, and the liver meridian and the organs it nourishes, such as the uterus, thyroid, and breasts, will stay healthy. If liver *qi* is slow or stagnant, metabolism is sluggish and there will be problems such as pain, fatigue, or nausea. If there is a long-standing *qi* constriction, toxic metabolites will build up, and you will have disease in these organs along the meridian. How well your *qi* moves very much determines your health.

Healthy Liver Metabolism: Keeping Hormones Safe

I find the liver infinitely exciting and miraculous, but it is not an organ much acclaimed in the Western world. Here, people pray for strong bones and a steadfast mind; odes are written about the tireless beating heart, but generally the liver garners little attention or appreciation. When I start talking about liver metabolism, most of my patients cringe or beg for mercy, saying, "Please, spare me the metabolic charts, and simply tell me what to do to make hormones safe." Those of you who feel this way should read the list below for some important ways to keep your liver happy and then move on to more exciting chapters. If you are intrigued to learn some liver science, continue reading beyond the list.

How to Keep Your Liver (and Your Hormones) Happy

- Avoid synthetic forms of any hormones, as the liver has a difficult time breaking them down. Natural bioidentical hormones are available in FDA-approved forms or can be custom-compounded.
- Use *transdermal* natural estradiol (described in chapter 9). This prevents high levels of hormones in the liver and reduces the risks of blood clots.
- Take a twenty-four-hour urine test each year to see how well your hormones are breaking down in your body. You want to make sure that you have plenty of 2-methoxyestrone and not too much 4-OH or 16-OH estrone. In the near future there will also be a urine test to measure quinones, the harmful hormone metabolites that predispose to breast cancer.
- Avoid or limit caffeine, alcohol, food additives, preservatives, trans fats, and multiple prescription medications. These all tax liver metabolism and predispose to stagnation.

- Eat organically as much as possible in order to minimize exposure to pesticides.
- Eat a diet rich in antioxidants (discussed in chapter 4). Four to five servings of colorful fruits each day is ideal.
- Avoid processed foods that lack nutrients and antioxidants.
- Eat a varied diet rich in legumes (beans, lentils), dark green leafy vegetables, cruciferous vegetables, and whole grains. In cultures where breast cancer is lowest, people eat a variety of cruciferous vegetables and legumes two to three times per day.
- Include flax meal (ground flaxseeds) in your diet. One to two tablespoons daily helps liver metabolism.
- Avoid dairy products that contain hormonal additives or growth factors, and cut down on dairy intake, particularly if you have signs of liver stagnation (breast pain, breast disease, PMS).
- If you are having liver stagnation symptoms, such as breast pain or PMS, use beta-sitosterol (500 to 800 mg/day), indole-3-carbinol (400 mg/day), Chinese herbal preparations, lipotropic complex (blend of herbs and nutrients to support liver health), or milk thistle (200 to 600 mg/day) to help hormone metabolism (see additional information at my Web site).
- Rotate antioxidants (use a bottle of one or two, and vary throughout the year) such as lipoic acid (200 mg/day), coenzyme Q10 (100 to 200 mg/day), vitamin C (1,000 to 2,000 mg/day), green tea extract, and NAC (N-acetylcysteine) (1,000 to 1,500 mg/day).
- Ensure that you are taking enough magnesium and B vitamins, particularly B_6, B_{12}, and folic acid.
- Request genetic testing to see if you have inherited problems breaking down estrogen, or problems with inflammation, clotting, or bone loss. Certain vitamins can be given to improve inherited metabolic problems. This testing is now available by specialty labs to detect SNPs (single nucleotide polymorphisms), referred to as "DNA snips," or genetic tendencies of how you metabolize estrogen (discussed later in this chapter).
- According to Chinese medicine, sour foods help the liver. Drinking lemon water (juice of one-half lemon in eight ounces of water in the morning and/or evening) helps liver flow and can improve fat metabolism. It has the added benefit of enhancing weight loss.

Some Science about Liver Metabolism

Understanding the science behind things can help to motivate you to eat and do the right things. For this reason I usually show my patients charts about how hormones break down inside them and how certain vitamins and foods can help hormones metabolize more safely.

As I've said, your liver is like a waste treatment facility and you don't want it to become overloaded. If your cells are overworked processing caffeine, alcohol, prescription drugs, or pesticides, then it may not do a very good job when it gets around to your hormones. This explains why women often complain of breast pain if they overuse caffeine, and why there is an increase in breast cancer in women who drink too much alcohol or are exposed to pesticides or other toxins.

We metabolize hormones in two phases, called simply Phase 1 and Phase 2, connected to each other by a metabolic pathway, or road, between metabolites. Vitamins, minerals, and enzymes regulate these pathways. An enzyme is a protein that drives a metabolic pathway. Think of enzymes as taxis that take you from the airport to your home. Some enzymes go slowly and some go very fast (genetics and nutrients determine their speed). For example, if there is a metabolic rush hour caused by too many medications and toxins to metabolize, a metabolic traffic jam may result. If this occurs, other metabolic routes or detours will develop and you may overproduce possibly harmful metabolites. Similarly, if you inherited a particularly slow enzyme pathway, or are deficient in B vitamins or other nutrients, an enzyme may not work well and the same problem can arise. Metabolic traffic jams result in toxic metabolites. Fortunately, your inherited enzymes can be helped by the right nutrients, thereby improving your hormone metabolism. As the Chinese observed, certain foods (green leafy vegetables, cruciferous plants, and sour foods) move liver *qi* and improve metabolism; other foods (fats, alcohol, caffeine, and dairy) cause the liver metabolism to stagnate. Over the long term, stagnation will give rise to disease along the liver meridian, that is, in the uterus, ovaries, breasts, and thyroid, and give rise to migraines. These diseases can be avoided with improvements in liver health.

When I treat liver problems, I use diet as well as herbal combinations and supplements to support Phase 1 and Phase 2 metabolism.

Supporting Phase 1 Metabolism

During Phase 1, hormones are chopped up into smaller, possibly danger-ous, pieces. These pieces, Phase 1 metabolites, are very active and, if oxi-dized (mixed with oxygen), can form free radicals. Free radicals cause many health problems such as heart disease, blood clots, cancer, arthri-tis, autoimmune disorders, and most problems associated with aging.

Our body naturally makes antioxidants to protect us from free-rad-ical damage, but our environment and aging reduce our antioxidant pool. Pesticides, synthetic hormones, cigarette smoke, pollution, and heavy metals (particularly lead and mercury) reduce our antioxidant levels and increase our risk of disease. Because our body's production of antioxidants declines as we age, we become increasingly susceptible to oxidation problems. For this reason, the problems of aging are pri-marily due to oxidation of free radicals. Cancer, heart disease, and dementia are largely the result of free-radical damage to our blood ves-sels and cells. This is where antioxidants are so important, particularly if you have inherited tendencies to make too many free radicals.

Because antioxidants work in combination with certain vitamins and minerals, eating foods naturally rich in antioxidants is the best way to protect yourself. But this isn't always easy to do. We live in a world of highly processed foods. Processing foods removes the natural blend of nutrients. Although many foods are now "fortified," often the way that they are fortified results in a food that is still not as healthy as what occurs naturally.

So what foods should you be eating? In general, those that are col-orful are highest in antioxidants. Berries (blackberries, strawberries, raspberries, blueberries, black currants, cherries), nuts (walnuts, sun-flower seeds), goji berries (also known in Chinatown as wolfberry), fruits (pomegranates, grapes, oranges, plums, pineapples, lemons, apri-cots, dates, kiwis, clementines, grapefruits), beans (pinto, soy), vegeta-bles (kale, red cabbage, peppers, parsley, artichokes, Brussels sprouts, spinach, red beets), cereals (barley, millet, oats, corn), and ginger are all very high in antioxidants. I encourage my patients to try to eat eight to nine servings of varied fruits, berries, and vegetables every day. Antiox-idants are discussed further in chapter 4. Because diet alone may not suffice, I usually recommend rotating antioxidants. Lipoic acid (100 mg twice daily), green tea extract, vitamin C (1,000 to 2,000 mg/day) and NAC (N-acetylcysteine, 1,000 to 1,500 mg/day) are some of the ones I recommend. Choose a bottle or two and take it for a month or so, then switch.

In addition to supporting antioxidant levels, our cytochrome P450 (the part of our liver where Phase 1 takes place) needs minerals such as iron, magnesium, selenium, and other trace minerals, as well as B vitamins, particularly riboflavin and niacin. Dark leafy greens are rich in these required minerals and vitamins, and cruciferous vegetables have chemicals known as indoles (discussed in chapter 4), which also help Phase 1. These vegetables are always part of any dietary liver cleanse and should be a regular part of your diet. Because so many women are low in B vitamins and magnesium, I usually supplement these as well with magnesium aspartate or magnesium glycinate (300 to 500 mg/day) and B complex (100 mg/day).

Improving Phase 2 Metabolism

In Phase 2 the breakdown products from Phase 1 are "glued" to substances so that the active pieces are not dangerous. This gluing together process is called *conjugation*. There are many conjugation possibilities, which are referred to as *pathways*. Two important pathways are described here to help you understand how your genetics, digestion, and eating habits affect your risk of breast cancer:

1. **Glucuronidation** attaches toxins to glucuronic acid. This is the primary way that women get rid of used estrogen (and most toxins in general). If you have an imbalance of bacteria in your gut (from antibiotics or insufficient digestive enzymes or parasites), harmful bacteria may produce a substance known as glucuronidase, which breaks the tie between estrogen and glucuronic acid and increases cancer risks (discussed below).

2. **Methylation** is one of the most important Phase 2 pathways that can help to prevent breast cancer and heart disease. How well you methylate (attach a carbon and hydrogen molecule CH_3, or methyl group, from the amino acid methionine), will determine how safely estrogen metabolizes in you. Poor methylation is

largely due to inherited genetic mutations, which can be detected from a simple blood test. You may also have problems methylating if you are low in vitamins B_{12}, B_6, and/or folic acid. You will be hearing a lot about methylation in the future, as methylation problems have been linked to cancer, dementia, and heart disease.

How do you know how well you are methylating? Well, if you have a strong family history of breast cancer or ovarian cancer, or you are prone to breast pain, be suspicious. In general, I recommend that all perimenopausal or estrogen-using menopausal women take a twenty-four-hour urine test every year to check their 2-methoxyestrone levels. Homocysteine levels are also informative. Homocysteine is an amino acid frequently measured by doctors to determine if you are at an increased risk for heart disease. High homocysteine levels indicate a problem with methylation.

What can you do about methylation problems? Most doctors prescribe vitamin combinations of vitamins B_6 (100 mg/day), B_{12} (1,000 mg/day), and folic acid (1 to 2 mg/day). If homocysteine levels remain elevated after two or three months of such therapy, I recommend polymorphic genetic testing (discussed at the end of this chapter) to see which enzymes are having trouble. Some women need very high doses (2 to 16 mg) of folinic acid or methylated folic acid, glutathione (from NAC, N-acetylcysteine), methionine, or betaine (trimethylglycine), or injections of high-dose methylated B_{12}. A doctor familiar with polymorphic testing will be able to guide you.

Bowels 101

In addition to liver metabolism, digestion is also key. Most hormones leave your body in your stool. For this reason, your bowels are important for good hormonal health. There is an established link between healthy gut function and cancer, particularly hormone cancers such as breast, prostate, and colon cancers. This is because an enzyme known as glucuronidase is produced by bacteria in your gut. Too much glucuronidase (from overgrowth of bacteria) can interfere with Phase 2 glucuronidation by dissolving the bond between estrogen and glucuronic acid. If this occurs, excess estrogen is reabsorbed from your gut. It's like opening your car window in a tunnel during rush hour. The fumes are free to enter your lungs and poison you. Antibiotics alter the bacteria in the gut and increase the likelihood of high glucuronidase activity. A Finnish study observed 10,000 women who took antibiotics chronically for recurrent urine infections and found that they had a 74 percent increased risk of breast cancer. You can measure glucuronidase in your stool.

How do you keep glucuronidase levels down? Your body produces calcium-d-glucarate to deactivate glucuronidase. Calcium-d-glucarate is also found in many fruits (particularly apples, oranges, and grapefruits) and vegetables (particularly cruciferous vegetables). Calcium-d-glucarate can also be taken as a supplement (500 to 1,500 mg/day).

To summarize, if your bowels are not working optimally, here are a few things that might help:

- You can have a digestive analysis to measure the amounts of digestive enzymes, glucuronidase, healthy bacteria, and unhealthy bacteria or yeast in your gut. Most specialty labs (see chapter 6) will provide herbal recommendations for overgrowth of bacteria or yeast and will measure the amount of glucuronidase in the stool. Organic acid tests from your urine can detect toxins from various bacteria and yeasts.
- Use digestive enzymes. Start with a broad-spectrum enzyme and add a specific enzyme if certain foods trigger symptoms. For example, use lipase if fats bother you, lactase if dairy is a problem, protease if proteins seem to cause symptoms, or something with bile if your gallbladder has been removed. You'll know it's right if your bowels improve.
- Chew your food well. This may sound so simple, but most people do not take the time to chew properly. Much digestion occurs in your mouth, and if foods are not well broken down, they can cause the gut to become rancid and fermented and you can become bloated with an overgrowth of bad bacteria. Food leaving your mouth should be pastelike.
- Use a probiotic, that is, living friendly bacteria such as acidophilus, bifidobacteria, or lactobacillus. This is particularly important if you have been on antibiotics. Take probiotics with

or without food, but keep them away from bowel-cleansing herbs, as these herbs could kill off the friendly bacteria you are trying to nurture.

- Flax meal (ground flaxseeds) is especially good for constipation and helps improve estrogen metabolism. One to two tablespoons daily is the recommended dose. Take more (two to four tablespoons) if you are constipated.
- Use the supplement calcium-d-glucarate (1,500 to 3,000 mg/day), particularly if your glucuronidase is high. You can measure glucuronidase levels in your stools with specialty lab testing.
- Basic herbs, such as pumpkin seeds, berberine, garlic, or caprylic acid, can clear up may bowel problems. Also, products with plant tannins can kill many unwanted bowel bacteria and yeast. You should notice improved bowel function while on the herbs. If not, you should do a digestive analysis or an organic acid test through specialty labs (listed in chapter 6). I recommend an herbal bowel cleanse to patients each spring, and certainly if there are digestive symptoms.
- Eat a healthy diet with plenty of whole grains, and four to eight varieties of fresh fruits and vegetables each day.

Genetics and Estrogen

We live in exciting medical times. You can determine from a simple blood test if you have inherited sluggish metabolic pathways that place you at risk for breast cancer, heart disease, or bone loss.

If one of your first-degree relatives has breast cancer, your risk of breast cancer increases twofold. This is because minor inherited genetic variations (genetic polymorphisms) cause your metabolism to suffer. Some of these gene defects cause methylation problems and limit your ability to make 2-methoxyestrone. If you have such an inherited tendency, specific vitamins and supplements (methylated B_{12}, high-dose folinic acid, I3C, NAC, and betaine) can improve and reduce your breast cancer risk. Polymorphic genetic tests can determine if you are prone to blood clots or excess 4-OH or 16-OH estrone production, if you have a tendency to low glutathione or other antioxidants, or if you are prone to inflammation in your vessels or a resistance to vitamin D.

This is truly preventive medicine. In the ideal world of the future, all women will understand their genetic tendencies and use hormones and supplements to correct their inherited shortcomings. At present such testing is not covered by insurance, but it is a once-in-a-lifetime test, which doesn't ever need to be repeated. This is fertile ground for research and important news for women with a history of breast cancer who are wondering why they developed cancer and what they can do to prevent it from recurring. I try to have all of my patients do polymorphic testing to better understand their metabolic weaknesses and risks.

Rarely, women require a test for two specific genes (known as BRCA1 and BRCA2 genes) that are closely linked to ovarian and breast cancer. Because BRCA genes are associated with a very high possibility of developing breast or ovarian cancer (about 80 percent probable), testing should be done with genetic counseling only when you have any of the following:

- A close family member with BRCA1 or BRCA2 genes.
- One or more close family members with breast cancer, ovarian cancer, or both. (Your chance of cancer is higher if either of these cancers occurred before age fifty, if several family members had these cancers, if the breast or ovarian cancer occurred in both breasts or ovaries, or if one family member had both cancers.)
- A male family member with breast cancer.
- A family member younger than age fifty with breast cancer, or who has ovarian cancer and is of Eastern European or Ashkenazi Jewish descent.

Summary: What You Need to Make Estrogen Safe

- Use natural transdermal estrogen, balanced with natural progesterone (transdermal or orally), for the symptoms of perimenopause and menopause.
- You need to have a healthy liver and digestion to safely process estrogen.
- For a healthy liver, you need a diet rich in cruciferous vegetables, green leafy vegetables, and fruits, and a clean environment,

avoiding exposure as much as possible to pesticides, preservatives, plastics, and food dyes. You also need to limit your alcohol and caffeine intake.

- For a healthy bowel, avoid overusing antibiotics, and if you do use them, replace friendly bacteria with probiotics. Consider bowel cleansing with herbs and/or testing for overgrowth of bacteria and yeast if your bowels are not moving regularly.
- Follow a diet high in antioxidants so that quinones won't form from 4-OH estrone. Consider rotating antioxidants throughout the year (discussed in chapter 4).
- Monitor hormone metabolites with a twenty-four-hour urine test each year.
- Maintain low levels of 4-OH estrone and 16-OH estrone to prevent overstimulation of the uterus and breast and avoid cancer-promoting quinones. If levels are high, supplement with I3C (400 mg/day).
- Maintain high 2-OH estrone levels.
- If your 2-methoxyestrone level is low (and/or your homocysteine level is high) take B vitamin combinations (100 mg of B_6, 1,000 mg of B_{12}, and 1 to 2 mg of folic acid) and I3C (400 mg) daily. If levels do not improve after two to three months, consult a doctor trained in testing and treating polymorphic genetic problems.
- If you have a family history of breast cancer or ovarian cancer, if you are prone to breast cysts, breast pain, or fibroids, or if you have poor metabolites, you should test for genetic polymorphisms. This will tell you what enzyme problems you have inherited and what supplements to use to improve your metabolic pathways.

Hormones and a Healthy Lifestyle

There is so much written about having a healthy lifestyle that we easily become numb to the recommendations—that is, until something goes wrong. If you or someone you love suddenly develops cancer or diabetes or has a stroke, you can't help but take a hard look at your lifestyle. We all sort of know innately when we are off, but we think, "Oh, I'll change that next month or come bathing suit weather." Before we know it, we are carrying an extra ten pounds and feeling frustrated, blaming our hormones or our too-busy life. But somewhere deep inside, we know how we got this way. Maybe it was by gradually eating out more and having an extra muffin or two. After all, the latest WHI report said that fat doesn't matter. Does it? It is just so confusing and easy to overindulge when we are tired and going fast, and the media keeps changing the tune.

Okay, I am not here to lecture you about slowing down—me a working mother of six, on the go twenty-four/seven, eating as best I can, always on the run. But I am here to explain how we get out of balance, and what happens in our body when we do and what the studies say and don't say about that. This chapter is about what happens when you don't do what we all know you should do. The great thing about your lifestyle is that it does affect your health—and it is never too late to make changes. The body is amazingly resilient, and we are very adaptable creatures most of the time.

Why We Care about Good Health

Most women fear breast cancer, but the reality is they should be more concerned about heart disease. Consider these facts:

- More women die from heart disease and stroke than do men.
- Heart disease is the leading cause of death in women, claiming a half-million lives annually.
- Heart disease kills twelve times as many women in the United States as breast cancer. More women die from heart disease than from breast, ovarian, and uterine cancers combined.
- Younger women—less than fifty years old—are twice as likely to die if they have a heart attack compared with men.
- One in ten women aged forty-five to sixty-four has some form of heart disease. This figure increases to one in five after age sixty-five.
- Most heart studies are conducted on men.
- Obesity is a leading risk factor for heart disease and cancer. Over 60 percent of all women are overweight. One-third of women who are overweight are obese. More men are overweight than women, but more women are obese.

The way things stand today, most of us women are going to die from heart disease and most of us will die in our late seventies or early eighties, overweight or obese. If we don't die of heart disease, we will most likely die from a stroke. If we get cancer, it will most likely be lung cancer. Only 3 percent of us will die from breast or colon cancer, about the same number of women who will die from diabetes.

That's the bad news. The good news is that you can change your statistics by changing your lifestyle.

The everyday choices that you make about what you do with your time, what you eat, and even what you decide to smear on your body affects your long-term health. Both heart disease and cancer are largely environmental, and by improving your lifestyle, you will reduce your risk of getting heart disease or cancer. Hitting the genetics lottery helps, but either way, avoiding hormones and fat is not the answer.

Both the Nurses' Health Study and the WHI study show that for women aged fifty to fifty-nine, using estrogen reduced heart disease, breast cancer, colon cancer, and the frequency of bone fractures. It did not show a reduction in heart disease for women over age sixty. Why? Because normally in women after age sixty-four (the median age for the WHI study was sixty-seven), heart disease doubles. Starting hormones at this age does not change that.

What you eat, think, do, and live near affects your risk of cancer and heart disease. Your lifestyle affects your hormone metabolism, fat metabolism, immune function, and sugar control. They are all interconnected. Fortunately, positive lifestyle changes help prevent heart disease, stroke, and cancer. You've heard it before, so I'll say this only once. Never doubt the importance of exercising regularly (at least three times a week) and eating well (four to six servings of fresh fruits and vegetables) each day. Take time out to enjoy yourself and your family. Avoid the fast lane of foods and activities and avoid pesticides, hidden hormones, and carcinogens in foods and cosmetics. It makes a difference. Here's why.

Diets Can Help or Hurt

Hippocrates advised us over 2,400 years ago: "Let food be your medicine, otherwise medicine will become your food." Unfortunately, many of us have not heeded this advice, and we are now consuming medications as if they were our food. Antacids, stomach acid blockers, sleep aids, antidepressants, and lipid-lowering drugs have become staples. When I was in medical school in the 1970s, only the elderly were on several medications; now, sadly, it has become the norm for many of us. What is worse, despite the rise in medication use, is that the health of our nation is deteriorating. The high incidence of depression, insomnia, digestive problems, and heart disease is a testament to this. Although we are certainly living longer, we seem to suffer more.

As I explained in chapter 3, foods affect our metabolism. Simply avoiding processed fast foods and eating a well-balanced diet of whole grains and fresh fruits and vegetables in moderation can cure most twentieth-century ills. Chinese medicine routinely uses food to treat all ailments. In my twenties, I sought the advice of a Chinese doctor who prescribed lamb and beef broth (in addition to herbs) to treat my fatigue and menstrual cramps. When I explained that I was vegetarian and didn't eat meat, he replied, "Meat is not food, it is medicine." I have included some meat in my diet ever since.

Eating the right foods can reduce your chances of heart disease, cancer, bone loss, constipation, irritable bowel syndrome, insomnia, high cholesterol, moodiness, fatigue, and more. Whole foods contain antioxidants, minerals, vitamins, and fiber as well as the nutrients needed for our cells to detox and metabolize. Unfortunately, much of what we are eating or being advised to eat is high in the wrong kinds of fats, high-fructose corn syrup, additives, preservatives, dyes, and empty calories. So let's look at fats—which seem to be in everyone's favorite foods.

Fats and Heart Disease

Fats taste great, but some fats are good and others are bad. Simply put, you need enough good fats, no bad fats, and enough antioxidants to prevent any fat from oxidizing and damaging your blood vessels. Heart disease was rare in our country before 1920, but by the mid-1950s it became the leading cause of death. We have been told that this increase is due to an increase in saturated fats, but from 1910 to 1970 saturated fat consumption plummeted as the use of vegetable oils, in the form of margarine, shortening, and refined oils, rose 400 percent. So, obviously, avoiding fat is not the answer. In fact, the Framingham study—the mother of all fat studies—proved just that. After forty years, those who consumed more cholesterol and saturated fat had lower cholesterol levels over time. It also showed that people who had a history of yo-yo dieting, with fluctuating weight, had a 70 percent increased risk of dying from heart disease. What this shows is that you need fats. If your fat intake is too low, your skin, nails, and hair will become dry and brittle, your moods will fall, your immune system will suffer, and you won't be able to think clearly. Fats are needed for our cells and hormones to function normally. Because all adrenal and sex hormones are made from cholesterol, a low-fat diet will worsen your hormone balance.

What's Good about Cholesterol

We have become a nation preoccupied with having low cholesterol. This is unfortunate, as cholesterol itself is not bad, and we women may actually need more than men for good health and long life. Cholesterol is a fat made by your liver that allows all cells to function normally. In addition to making all cell membranes, cholesterol makes all of your adrenal and sex hormones as well as vitamin D and digestive juices (bile) needed to digest fats. People who have diets that are too low in fat suffer from immune problems, depression, bone loss, digestive complaints, and more.

Cholesterol made by your liver needs to be carried to cells, and it does so linked to either LDL (bad cholesterol) or HDL (good cholesterol). There are actually no good or bad cholesterols, but too much LDL can become oxidized, causing damage to vessels, and causing plaque to form in your blood vessels, leading to hardening of the arteries (atherosclerosis). HDL is not damaging and seems to help out the body by carrying LDL back to the liver. It may also help to remove plaque from blood vessels. Lipoprotein-a is a genetic variation of LDL. It is not clear how, but this type of LDL seems to worsen LDL damage. Triglycerides are a form of fat also made by your body that can cause damage if oxidized. All forms of fat, when they become oxidized, can damage vessels and cause inflammation. It is oxidation and inflammation, not the fats, that lead to heart attacks and strokes. It is believed that much of the effectiveness of many lipid-lowering drugs is their ability to reduce inflammation, not fat.

Everyone needs fat in their diet, but how much you need and how much your body makes are two different things. Our liver produces most of the cholesterol in our bodies; our diet contributes only about 4 percent. When your diet is low in cholesterol, your liver is programmed to make more. This is one reason that low-cholesterol diets don't lower cholesterol long-term. Healthy cholesterol levels may actually vary in men and women. What is good for men may not be for women. Women have a higher concentration of body fat and a higher hormonal need than men. We may require higher levels of cholesterol for our hormones. No studies to date using drugs or diet to lower cholesterol in normal women have shown a lower incidence of heart disease. High cholesterol has been shown to be a predictor of heart disease in men, but high cholesterol has never been shown to increase the risk of heart disease in normal women. This is why most cholesterol studies involve men only. Predictors of heart disease in women have been low HDL and low estradiol. Studies have shown that women over age fifty who had a low cholesterol level actually had an increased risk of death and an increase in depression, anxiety, and cancer. Other studies have shown an increase in brain hemorrhage in both men and women with very low cholesterol levels.

Despite these findings, current recommendations for both men and women are the same, and recommendations are now coming out that support reducing cholesterol to even lower levels, below what is normally found in men and women naturally. This is not good advice for a normal, healthy woman who needs adequate cholesterol for her hormone production. Now, I am not saying don't ever treat a very high cholesterol level. If you are diabetic or have a history of heart disease, maintaining a normal cholesterol level is important and has been shown to be helpful. But if you don't have these problems, recognize that a high cholesterol level is not a disease, it is a symptom of an imbalance. If your thyroid function or estrogen levels are low, your cholesterol will be high. In women, avoiding cholesterol and fat are clearly not the answer.

Despite low-cholesterol diets and cholesterol-lowering drugs, both men and women have experienced an increase in heart disease. Although there have been fewer deaths from heart disease in men, there has been a steady increase in congestive heart failure and an unchanged incidence of heart attacks. There have been some recent reports that the incidence of heart attacks is increasing in women, as our consumption of eggs, butter, and animal fats has fallen. Statins—drugs that lower cholesterol—have been shown to reduce heart attacks from recurring but not from happening. A study published in the *American Journal of Cardiology* in 2003 showed that the amount of arterial disease (plaque) was not different in groups given high doses of statin drugs (lowering the cholesterol to one-half the normal value), compared with patients on low-dose statins (maintaining low-normal levels of cholesterol). Both groups had more plaque after one year.

What's the Problem with Fat?

So if cholesterol isn't the problem, how much and what kinds of fats can we safely eat? Some fats are better than others, and some fats should be avoided altogether. The Nurses' Health Study (NHS), discussed in chapter 3, showed that the types of fats women eat matter more than the amount. The most harmful fats were trans fats and hydrogenated fats. Trans fats are formed when liquid vegetable oils go through a chemical process called hydrogenation. Hydrogen added to fat makes it more solid. Trans fats are not normally found in nature, and our bodies have a hard time metabolizing them. (Sound familiar? I liken this to the difference between synthetic and natural hormones.) Industry loves trans fats because products made with them never seem to go bad (it seems bacteria can't handle them, either). In the NHS study, 80,000 women aged thirty-four to fifty-nine were followed over fourteen years, and it was shown that replacing saturated and trans fats with unhydrogenated fats was more effective in reducing heart disease than cutting down on overall fat intake. Using natural fats appears to help prevent heart disease.

What about the WHI study on fats? Well, the media's misunderstanding of the findings seems to have taken us a giant step back in time, with headlines proclaiming "Low-Fat Diets Don't Make a Difference." The WHI study followed roughly 49,000 women, aged fifty to seventy-nine, for an average of eight years. It examined the incidence of heart disease and cancer rates in women on a low-fat diet, compared with women eating normally. All groups began by eating a diet with fat amounting to 35 to 38 percent of their total calorie intake. The low-fat group was asked to lower their fat intake to 20 percent of their total calories, but this was never achieved. At the end of the first year, the low-fat group was eating fat at a rate of 24 percent of their total calories, and by the sixth year this had expanded to 29 percent. The comparison group averaged 35 percent at the end of one year and 38 percent at the end of the sixth year. The low-fat group was also asked to increase their consumption of fruit, vegetables, and grains, but the investigators admitted that "the differences in fruit and vegetable intakes were modest." In other words, the diets of the two groups were not vastly different. Despite this, there were reductions in heart disease and colonic polyps and adenomas (precursors of colon cancer) in the low-fat group and there was a 9 percent reduction in breast cancer, as well. But because statistical wizards deemed this "insignificant," it was dismissed as a negative study in the press, creating confusion for the average woman just trying to do the right thing.

Critics of the WHI fat study comment on the fact that this study was originally designed to look at cancer rates only, and did not differentiate between "good fats" found in fish, nuts, and vegetable oils and "bad fats" such as saturated fats and trans fats. This study, like the NHS study, showed that just reducing total fat didn't reduce heart disease. Prior studies reporting more striking results used more stringent diets and controlled for fat types.

Good Fat

Now we all realize that trans fats are bad, and many states are actually moving to ban their use, but what fats are good? Essential fatty acids are fats that our body is unable to make on its own. There are two types: omega-3 and omega-6. Omega-3 fatty acids are most important, as they bring balance to our hormones, reduce inflammation, regulate our blood sugar, prevent blood clotting, keep our cholesterol and triglycerides in balance, relax our blood vessels, and make our cells healthy and resilient. Omega-3 fats are found in fish oil, olive oil, flaxseeds, pumpkin seeds, sunflower seeds, and some organ meats. The most important omega-3 fats are EPA (eicosapentaenoic acid) and DHA (docosahexaenoic acid), both made from alpha linoleic acid. In order to make DHA and EPA, your body must have sufficient vitamin B_6, vitamin B_3, vitamin C, magnesium, and zinc. Many medications (oral contraceptives, oral estrogen) and conditions (excess stress, infection, cancer) cause a deficiency of such vitamins, which can lead to low levels of omega-3. Symptoms of inadequate omega-3 are mood swings, depression, dry skin, digestive upset, and immune problems.

Until the modern age, we humans routinely ate a diet of nearly equal omega-3 and omega-6 oils, naturally. Since the industrial revolution and the advent of vegetable oils, our diets have gradually changed. Living busy lives dependent upon easy-to-prepare, easy-to-pick-up fast foods, we have developed diets that are typically high in omega-6 and low in omega-3 (often twenty to fifty times more omega-6 than omega-3). Consequently, as our diets have changed, disease patterns have shifted toward more depression, hormone imbalance, and diseases of inflammation, including a high incidence of autoimmune diseases, particularly in women. It is no wonder that antidepressants have now surpassed lipid-lowering drugs as the most frequently prescribed medications.

In order to absorb fatty acids from your food, your digestion must work properly, and for that you need enough bile and digestive enzymes. Sadly, many women whom I see with bone loss have digestive problems and are unable to absorb fats and fat-soluble vitamins (vitamins A, D, E, and K). In addition to having deficient hormones, these women have mood problems (from lack of omega-3 fatty acids) as well as difficulty making new bone. Specialty lab tests can measure your digestive enzymes and the fat content of your stool to see if this is a problem. If so, lipase and bile supplements can be added to help you absorb essential fats. Many women with bone loss are put on medications when they in fact need hormones, lipase, magnesium, trace minerals, and vitamins B_3 (niacin), B_6, D, E, and K.

Recommendations to Reduce Heart Disease

- Support estrogen in the first ten years of menopause and ensure that your thyroid and adrenal hormones are working optimally.
- Eat a diet rich in antioxidants (ideally two to four fresh, multicolored fruits and two to four fresh, multicolored vegetables each day) and/or supplement your diet with antioxidants.
- Avoid trans fats as much as possible and limit saturated fats to 10 percent of your total calories. Read labels on food packaging and avoid prepared cookies, crackers, breads, and fried fast foods that contain trans fats or hydrogenated oil. Choose instead whole-grain, high-fiber foods.
- Eat adequate omega-3 fatty acids (from fish, nuts, beans, olive oil) or supplement with omega-3 fatty acids by rotating your consumption of fish, flax, and EPA/DHA oils. Rotate these with

borage and evening primrose oils that provide a natural blend of omega-3 and omega-6, particularly helpful to hormone balance.
- Exercise thirty minutes each day, ideally.
- Maintain a normal weight.

Cancer and Diet

Most people develop cancer from an environmental exposure affecting a genetic tendency. We also know that such genetic tendencies can be improved by the foods we eat.

Studies done on Asian populations have really helped to clarify the role of diet and environment on cancer. Asians and Asian Americans have the lowest risk of breast cancer compared with any other ethnic group. In 1993, a study showed that Asian American women born in the West had a 60 percent higher incidence of breast cancer than Asian Americans born in the East. Furthermore, Asian American women with three or four grandparents born in the West had a 50 percent higher risk than those women with all grandparents born in the East. Studies also show that immigrants who lived in the West for ten years or more had an 80 percent higher risk of developing cancer than recent immigrants. This clearly shows that diet, environment, and lifestyle trump genetics in reducing the risk of breast cancer.

Fat and Breast Cancer

Numerous studies have linked an increased incidence of breast cancer in women with diets high in animal fat and dairy (red meat, cheese, ice cream. and butter). But is it the fat content or something else? There are three reasons to explain such a trend: (1) hidden hormones in meats and dairy; (2) weight gain on such diets; and (3) how the meats are prepared.

1. Hidden hormones in meat and dairy are a problem. Red meat and dairy contain growth hormones, sex hormones, and antibiotics. (Hormone use is prohibited in poultry and pork.) It is estimated that 90 percent of U.S. livestock is injected with some form of hormone and up to 30 percent of dairy cows receive hormones. In addition, pollutants and pesticides in the animals'

food supply (which then becomes stored in the animals' fat) might trigger breast cancer.

2. Women who eat high-fat foods tend to be overweight, and overweight women produce more estrogen and have a higher rate of breast cancer. So is it what's in the fat or what the fat does? Fat is active. It is constantly producing hormones and inflammatory proteins. Unfortunately, fat tends to make estrone, and a form of estrogen, which is associated with breast cancer.

3. The way you cook your meat plays a role, too. Charcoal broiling or high-heat grilling can produce substances known to increase the incidence of breast cancer.

Foods and Estrogen Metabolism

As you saw in chapter 3, estrogen is complicated when it breaks down, but how it breaks down helps to determine your risk for cancer. Both our environment and our genes affect our metabolism of estrogen. Food can greatly affect this.

There are four groups of foods that can improve how you break down estrogen: (1) cruciferous vegetables (I3C foods); (2) phytoestrogens, of which there are three types—isoflavones (such as soy), lignans (or flax meal), and coumestans (found in legumes); (3) phytosterols; and (4) antioxidant-rich foods.

Cruciferous Vegetables

Your mother always told you to eat your Brussels sprouts and broccoli, but she probably didn't really know why. Cruciferous vegetables are medicinal and can alter how estrogen is broken down and reduce your chances of developing breast cancer. The Asian diet is very high in cruciferous vegetables and this most likely explains the low rate of breast cancer found in Asians, particularly Asians eating the traditional Asian diet of stir-fried vegetables and small amounts of animal protein. What is it about cruciferous vegetables? It is all about indole-3-carbinol, or I3C.

I3C is a plant substance (known as an indole) that helps convert estrogen into the good metabolites (2-OH estrones) instead of the bad metabolites (16-OH or 4-OH estrones) associated with cancer. I3C has been shown to prevent breast cancer cells from growing and can also help to regulate estrogen receptors. If you have a genetic polymorphism or a strong family history of breast cancer, I3C can help you make more of the beneficial 2-OH estrones and fewer 16-OH estrones. I3C converts into DIM (diindolylmethane) in your digestive tract. Both I3C and DIM improve estrogen metabolites and are available as suppplements. Because DIM is less expensive and doesn't require stomach acid to work, it is often touted as the preferred supplement. However, DIM doesn't have the anticancer properties or the estrogen-receptor effects that I3C does. I recommend using 400 mg daily of I3C (equivalent to eating one half of a head of cabbage). I often prescribe this with a low dose of betaine hydrochloride, which ensures acid to make DIM and helps methylation.

Ideally, your diet should contain a variety of cruciferous vegetables, eaten at least twice daily. Most Americans eat none or one serving of cruciferous vegetables daily; the typical Asian diet consumes four or more servings per day. If you are following your estrogen metabolites with a twenty-four-hour urine test, you will actually see a shift in your estrogens for the better when you increase your intake of cruciferous veggies.

Vegetables high in I3C
- Broccoli, cauliflower
- Bok choy (there are several varieties)
- Chinese cabbage
- Watercress
- Rapini, broccolini
- Red, white, and Savoy cabbage
- Brussels sprouts
- Kale, kohlrabi
- Collard greens, mustard greens

I encourage my patients to cook extra cruciferous vegetables at dinner, and add them to their soup, salad, or rice for lunch. Most of the vegetables listed above can be quickly stir-fried alone or in combination. The ideal is to eat two servings twice daily. If you simply can't tolerate these vegetables, use I3C. If you are on medications to lower your stomach acid, you may want to use DIM with I3C. No one yet knows the ideal amount of 2-OH estrone, but we do know that women with breast cancer have a ratio of 2-OH estrone to 16-OH estrone of less than two to one. The current recommendation is a ratio that is greater than two to one (determined by twenty-four-hour urine tests).

Phytoestrogens

Most hormones are made from cholesterol, and some plants contain compounds that are similar in shape to cholesterol and act like hormones in your body. If a plant substance has the same chemical shape as estrogen, it is called a phytoestrogen. In low doses, phytoestrogens can act like estrogen and stimulate cells, but in high doses they they can block estrogen effects. To complicate matters, not all phytoestrogens are the same. There is confusion about the risk of phytoestrogens in women with a history of breast cancer. Some studies have found benefits, others haven't. Although most cancer specialists recommend that women with a history of breast cancer limit their phytoestrogen intake, no studies have shown an increase in breast cancer with moderate or high phytoestrogen diets. However, studies abound showing cancer-protective effects of phytoestrogens. I believe moderation in all things; don't overindulge in any treatment.

Phytoestrogens are food and can be divided into three types: isoflavones, lignans, and coumestans.

1. **Isoflavones**   During menopause, when estrogen is lowest, isoflavones have been found helpful to reduce hot flashes, increase bone density, reduce heart disease, and possibly reduce cancer. Soy is the most studied isoflavone because it has the highest phytoestrogen content of all foods. It can do a lot of good for women, but there are problems if soy is used excessively. If you are still cycling and making estrogen, too much soy can stimulate your breast cells, causing breast pain and worsening fibrocystic breasts. Most Asian diets are lower in soy than many U.S. diets. Asians consume about a quarter to a half cup per day, while with the recent soy enthusiasm, many women in North America are consuming double or triple this amount. I see many women who complain of breast tenderness on diets with excess soy, and for this reason I recommend not using more than about one to two

cups of soy products daily, less if you are cycling and suffer from breast disease.

The way your soy is prepared matters. Fermented soy products are the best because they don't contain phytates or digestion inhibitors and they are less stimulating to the breast. So instead of pouring soy milk over your cornflakes or mixing it in your fruit smoothies, use fermented soy products such as tempeh (good in soups or stews) and season your foods with fermented soy sauce. Try drinking miso soup, which is easily made from miso paste. Unfermented soy products, such as soy milk and tofu, are less desirable because they contain phytates and enzyme inhibitors that can interfere with your digestion and thyroid function. Phytates bind minerals such as iron, zinc, and calcium, which can also worsen bone health and thyroid function. Digestion inhibitors in unfermented soy can reduce many of the nutrients you absorb from your food and can cause excess gas or indigestion.

2. **Lignans**   Lignans are a group of phytoestrogens that are converted by "good" bacteria in our gut into substances that improve estrogen metabolism. Lignans are found in a wide variety of foods, including seeds, whole grains, and legumes, but the highest amounts by far are found in flax seeds.

LIGNAN CONTENT OF FOODS

FOOD	SERVING	TOTAL LIGNAN (MG)
Ground flaxseeds	1 oz.	85.5
Sesame seeds	1 oz.	11.2
Kale	½ cup chopped	0.8
Broccoli	½ cup chopped	0.6
Apricots	½ cup sliced	0.4
Cabbage	½ cup chopped	0.3
Brussels sprouts	½ cup chopped	0.3
Strawberries	½ cup chopped	0.3
Strawberries	¼ cup sliced	0.2
Tofu	½ block (4 oz.)	0.2
Dark rye bread	1 slice	0.1

Flax is one of the most ancient grains, and the early Greeks believed it was a blessed plant that could bring good fortune, restore health, and protect against witchcraft. Flax meal (ground flaxseeds) used to be part of our diets for thousands of years, until the advent of processed flours. Flax meal is high in lignans and can reduce your risk of hormone cancers by improving estrogen metabolism, lowering cholesterol, and regulating your digestion. Bacteria in your gut convert lignans into two substances, enterodiol and enterolactone. Studies have shown that high levels of these substances are associated with a lower incidence of osteoporosis, heart disease, and breast, uterine, and ovarian cancer. Women who have taken antibiotics chronically have lower levels of these lignan substances because antibiotics destroy all bacteria, good and bad, so they have less of the "good" bacteria in their bowels to convert lignan.

As flax consumption has decreased in industrialized countries, cancer, heart disease, and constipation have risen. But flaxseeds, flax meal, and flax oil are making a comeback. Whole flaxseeds help with constipation, but because these seeds are so difficult to digest, flaxseeds typically pass through us undigested and the lignan quality is lost. Flax oil is the highest food source for omega-3 fatty acids and is great for your mood, skin, hair, nails, and digestion; but because lignans are not oil-soluble, flax oil is not very effective for helping your estrogen metabolize better. For improved estrogen metabolism, you really need to eat ground flaxseeds.

You can grind flaxseeds in a coffee grinder or simply buy flax meal, available in most health food stores. A 2004 study published in the *Clinical Journal of Nutrition* showed that when women ate a muffin with 25 grams of flax meal daily (a little less than one ounce) they had an improved ratio of 2-OH to 16-OH estrogen metabolites. I recommend that women who are on hormone support, or have a history of breast cancer or a strong family history of breast cancer, use one to two tablespoons of ground flaxseeds per day for lignan benefits. Flax meal is good in smoothies, cereals, oatmeal, salads, and soups; mixed with juice (apricot juice is my favorite) or lemon water; or baked in muffins or bread.

3. **Coumestans**   Coumestans are the least studied of all phytoestrogens, but research has shown some cancer-preventing effects. Coumestans are found in legumes such as black beans, black-eyed peas, garbanzo beans, navy beans, pinto beans, lima beans, and kidney beans, as well as in alfalfa sprouts. They are also found in honey bush tea and green rooibos tea (both African teas). As you read in chapter 3, legumes support Phase 1 and 2 metabolism in the liver. Beans are a major food source in most of the world, but have somehow been forgotten in most North American diets. Beans are rich sources of antioxidants, fiber, trace minerals, and phytoestrogens, and they should be a regular part of your diet.

Phytosterols

You've probably never heard of them, but phytosterols are plant compounds that can improve estrogen metabolism, lower cholesterol absorption from your food, and lower cholesterol production in your liver. I use them a lot in my practice in lieu of Lipitor or other lipid-lowering medications and if women are having breast tenderness.

Sitosterols, a type of phytosterol, are found in all plant foods, particularly wheat germ, soybeans, corn oil, peanuts, wheat bran, and rye. Other foods that contain high levels of sitosterol are avocados, grape leaves, olive oil, corn oil, lentils, and even baking chocolate. Nuts such as macadamia nuts, peanuts, hazelnuts, walnuts, pecans, and almonds are also good sources of phytosterols. Wheat germ and sesame seeds contain the highest amounts of phytosterols (400 mg/100 gm of nuts), and pistachios and sunflower kernels have the next highest (280 mg/100 gm of nuts).

In Europe beta-sitosterol, a form of phytosterol, is prescribed to alleviate breast tenderness, improve liver function, prevent gallstone formation, lower cholesterol, and improve estrogen metabolism in women and men (it helps the symptoms of prostate enlargement). Beta-sitosterol also plays a role in weight loss, since it enhances fat metabolism. The typical North American diet used to be higher in beta-sitosterol, but with increased consumption of processed foods and genetically modified foods, our diet has become relatively deficient. I have no doubt that this deficiency has contributed to the rise in both heart disease and cancer.

I recommend supplementing your diet with beta-sitosterol, particularly if you are a woman with breast tenderness, fibrocystic breast disease, or high cholesterol. I have most of my patients use a beta-sitosterol supplement (600 to 800 mg/day) for three to four months, then take a break for two to three months, and repeat. For high lipids I recommend similar doses long-term, while trying to improve diet and liver function (with herbs and acupuncture). I have had great success with this.

Antioxidants

Antioxidants have gained much popularity for preventing skin wrinkles, but from reading chapter 3, you now know that antioxidants also protect us from the possible damaging effects of free radicals, particularly 4-OH estrone, which when oxidized forms a strong breast cancer–promoting quinone.

Fresh fruits and vegetables are rich in antioxidants such as carotene and vitamins C, A, and E. Antioxidants have been proven protective against many cancers, including lung, colon, breast, prostate, and ovarian cancer. In general, the more colorful the food you eat, the higher its antioxidant content will be. Cooking and microwaving lower the amount of antioxidants in your foods, so fresh is always best. Berries, pomegranates, sunflower seeds, and walnuts are foods with some of the highest antioxidant content. All citrus fruits, including oranges, pineapples, kiwi fruits, prunes, and dates, are also very good sources. Vegetables high in antioxidants include kale, red cabbage, red and green peppers, parsley, artichokes, Brussels sprouts, and spinach. Roots such as ginger and red beets are also great. Even grains contain antioxidants, particularly barley, corn, oats, and millet. Legumes such as black beans, lentils, broad beans, pinto beans, and other beans are high in antioxidants as well (generally, the darker the bean, the richer its antioxidant value).

If you are eating a well-balanced diet with three to four servings of vegetables and two to three fruit servings daily, and you are drinking green tea in place of coffee, you will probably be well protected. If you are not eating in this way, supplementing antioxidants may be important to reduce your cancer and heart disease risk. But be careful not to take the same multivitamin and/or antioxidants for months or years on end, as this may cause some nutrients to rise to unnatural levels. When I measure vitamins and antioxidants in my patients, there are often excessive levels of some antioxidants, particularly beta-carotene, because many foods are fortified with beta-carotene and it is in most multivitamins. For this reason, I recommend rotating vitamins and antioxidants.

Rotating supplements is important to avoid excessive dosing. Rotation is, after all, how we as cave dwellers received our nutrition. We ate what we scavenged. As seasons changed so did the foods we ate, thereby rotating our antioxidants and other nutrients. Chinese medicine recommends rotating foods to fit the season. For my patients who can't or won't stick to a well-balanced diet, I provide the following list of antioxidants and ask that they pick one or two to rotate every two to three months.

- Vitamin E 400 U daily (Use a mixed source with alpha and gamma tocopherol.)
- Selenium 200 mcg daily
- Lipoic acid 100 to 300 mg/day
- Vitamin C 1,000 to 2,000 mg/day
- Green tea extract (Doses vary with extract strength, usually 1 to 2 capsules daily.)
- NAC (N-acetylcysteine) 500 to 1500 mg/day (N-acetylcysteine is used to raise glutathione levels naturally. Glutathione is important for detoxifying dangerous substances in our liver. Glutathione is not absorbed from the digestive tract, so NAC is one of the only ways to raise glutathione inside the body safely. NAC is used to counter the effects of heavy metals and other toxins from pollution and chemical exposures.)
- CoQ10 100 to 200 mg/day (It is very important to use this supplement if you are on a statin lipid-lowering medication.)

There are specialty labs that can measure your vitamins and antioxidant levels to tailor-make your replacement. These are listed in chapter 6. Better yet, eat your fresh fruits and vegetables. If you eat plenty of what is in season, you will naturally rotate your nutrients. My Web site currently offers seasonally rotated multivitamins and antioxidants.

Coffee and Green Tea

Green tea is the most popular tea in China and Japan, where the lowest breast cancer rates are found. There are many health-promoting properties to green tea, and thousands of published studies verifying its benefits. Tea is generally high in antioxidants, but green is highest. Green tea is the least processed of all teas (green tea leaves are simply steamed). Oolong tea has some antioxidant effect, but lower levels than green tea, and black tea has the lowest levels of the three. White tea is similar to green tea (not fermented or processed), but the tea leaves are picked before the leaves open fully.

Green tea has been shown to lower risks of bacterial and viral infections, heart disease, stroke, cancer, gum disease, and even bone loss. Hundreds of studies have reported the benefits of green tea, which include reduced heart disease, lower triglycerides, less blood clotting, and lowered breast, ovarian, and prostate cancer, with less recurrence of cancer as well. It has been touted as a weight loss tool because it supports leptin, the hormone that controls our appetite and helps us burn fat. Studies published in 2005 in the *Archives of Internal Medicine* showed that in Swedish women aged forty to seventy-six years, there was a 24 percent lower risk of ovarian cancer in women who drank one cup of green tea daily; if they consumed two or more cups daily, their risk fell by 46 percent, compared with non–tea drinkers.

Clearly, the benefits of green tea increase with the amount of tea imbibed, but this might be too much caffeine or liquids for the average woman. Green tea contains about 15 mg of caffeine per cup. For this reason there are many green tea extracts available, which provide the benefits without the caffeine. (If you are sensitive to caffeine, you can simply steep the tea for a short time, as the caffeine is released faster, within thirty to sixty seconds. Pour off this water, then resteep your tea to obtain the antioxidants. This usually requires two to four minutes.) The substances that seem to work the magic in green tea are known as catechins, which make up about 30 percent of the dry weight of green tea leaves. The most active catechin is EGCG (epigallocatechin gallate), which I mention because when looking at green tea extracts, the higher the EGCG content, the more potent the product. So get your caffeine from green tea, not coffee.

Okay, now let me rant a bit about coffee. I am not a coffee drinker but I do realize that most of this country is fueled by it. Both coffee and tea contain antioxidants, but the coffee-roasting process destroys almost all of the antioxidant benefits. Very high temperatures are needed to process coffee, creating rancid oils and free radicals such as lipid peroxides, which can damage blood vessels and lower your antioxidant levels. No studies have shown an increased risk of breast cancer from caffeine, but coffee does have an adverse affect on liver metabolism in general.

Chinese medicine teaches that symptoms such as PMS, irritability, headache, and nausea are typically from stagnation or poor flow of energy through the liver meridian, and caffeine and alcohol are often cited as a common cause of liver stagnation. In the West, there is debate in the medical literature about this. Most texts simply take the position that "the cause of fibrocystic breast disease (FBD) remains unclear" and studies have been conflicting. I believe that there are many causes (including estrogen excess, progesterone deficiency, iodine deficiency, and low thyroid function), but no matter what the cause, the estrogen in the breast is not breaking down healthfully. I do advise avoiding caffeine and alcohol, for that matter, to improve hormone metabolism.

Caffeine can also have other ill effects. It can combine with stomach acid to form a toxin, caffeine hydrochloride, which causes the body to secrete excess bile from the liver. (This increase in bile is why caffeine stimulates bowel movements.) Over time, excess bile loss can deplete many of your essential liver nutrients. There is some caffeine in green tea, but much less than in other teas or coffee, and the pharmacologic action of green tea caffeine actually enhances liver function rather than depletes it. The green tea effect is a calm alertness, rather than the more anxious or irritable mood often seen with caffeine from coffee.

Don't think that you can avoid the problem with decaf. Decaffeinated coffee may be more harmful to the liver, as the process used to decaffeinate coffee beans usually uses large amounts of toxic chemicals, such as formaldehyde and trichloroethylene, which is used as a degreasing agent in the metal industry and as a solvent in dry cleaning. For this reason I recommend using organic decaffeinated blends.

Beverage	Caffeine content (mg)
Coffee, brewed (8 oz.)	80–135
Espresso (2 oz.)	40–60
Tea, black brewed (8 oz.)	45
Tea, green (8 oz.)	15–20
Tea, white (8 oz.)	15
Hot chocolate (8 oz.)	14
Coffee, decaf (8 oz.)	2–4
Pepsi-Cola (8 oz.)	55
Snapple sweet tea (8 oz.)	12

Alcohol

Multiple studies have confirmed that drinking more than two glasses of alcohol per day, whether it's beer, wine, or hard liquor, will increase your risk of breast cancer by roughly 40 percent. The results from a study of more than 150,000 women from around the world have shown that the more alcohol you drink, the greater your risk. The studies report the risks this way: If one hundred women drink two drinks per day, when they reach the age of eighty, there will be two more women with breast cancer than you would normally expect. Now, if these women drink six drinks per day, it increases to five more cases. These are higher risks than were seen in the WHI study, which showed only eight new cases of breast cancer per ten thousand women. Despite such high results, you haven't heard much press hysteria discouraging the use of alcohol the same way that hormone use has been discouraged. Some studies have shown that supplementing with folate can help to reduce this risk.

Exercise

A WHI cohort study showed that women who exercised the equivalent of brisk walking for 1.25 to 2.5 hours per week had an 18 percent reduction in the risk of breast cancer. This reduction increased further as physical activity increased, though not substantially. The reduction was less pronounced when a woman was overweight. Exercise has also been shown to improve survival rates after a diagnosis of breast cancer. I recommend that all of my patients exercise at least three times each week with thirty or more minutes of an aerobic session, and weight training twice weekly for bone health.

Environmental Pollutants

In the 1950s, one woman in twenty was likely to develop breast cancer; currently, one in nine is at risk. Exposure to environmental toxins is believed responsible for as much as 75 percent of all breast cancers. Although the death rate from breast cancer has fallen in the last decade (believed to be due to earlier diagnosis), breast cancer in the United States rose 1 percent each year from 1950 until 1998, when rates began to fall by 1 to 2 percent per year. There was a further, more significant drop in 2002 to 2003, when the rates of breast cancer suddenly fell by 7.2 percent. In fall 2006 this drop in breast cancer was publicized, but sadly, it was attributed to a fall in hormone use, which is misleading. The dramatic fall was in the use of *synthetic* hormones Premarin and Provera, the synthetic hormones used in the WHI study, not *all* hormones. Estrogen was not shown to be carcinogenic in the study, but Provera was implicated.

A similar drop in breast cancer was seen in Israel after pesticides were banned in dairy products in 1978. This was the first clear evidence of environmental toxins causing breast cancer. There are many confirmed and suspected culprits. Xenoestrogens are chemicals found in the environment from pesticides or chemical fertilizers. They behave like estrogen in the body and have been linked to breast and prostate cancer. Many pesticides have been found in foods. In Israel, the three organochlorine pesticides banned (lindane, DDT, and BHC, or benzene hexachloride) were contaminating milk and dairy foods. DDT has since been banned in the United States, but it is still used overseas and can be found in many imported meats. DDT is converted in the body into DDE, which remains in the body for decades and has been linked to breast cancer.

Examples of other common xenoestrogens are dioxin plastics, chlorinated products, and polycyclic aromatic hydrocarbons, which are derived from gasoline and oil combustion and found in cigarette smoke and charbroiled meats. They are literally everywhere—in our plastics, food wraps, water, air, spermicides, nail polish, and vaginal lubricants.

As if these kinds of environmental exposure were not enough, we women may be smearing carcinogens on our bodies every day unknowingly. Nearly all skin products, deodorants, and cosmetics contain preservatives, known as parabens, that have been linked to breast cancer. Methylparaben has been shown to enter the skin and is concentrated in our fat cells. In 1998 it was found that parabens can behave like estrogen, and studies since have shown that parabens cause breast cancer in rats. A British study in 2004 showed high levels of methylparaben in breast cancer cells. Though these studies are not definitive, there is growing concern that parabens may be linked to breast cancer, which would have enormous implications for the cosmetic industry.

Plastics contain products such as bisphenol-A, which was originally developed as a synthetic estrogen and is in plastic bottles used for drinking water, baby bottles, food wraps, and dental composites. Studies have shown that heating plastic wrap with foods containing oil or fats raises the xenoestrogen content of the food.

Conclusion

In summary, here are some ways to improve your lifestyle:

- Exercise regularly three to four times each week.
- Maintain a normal body weight.
- Avoid excess alcohol (ideally limit to two or three drinks per week).
- Eat two to four servings of cruciferous vegetables daily, and if you have a family history of breast cancer, take I3C (400 mg/day) and monitor your metabolites.
- Aim to eat four to five servings of fresh vegetables and two to four servings of fresh fruits daily. The more colorful foods are high in antioxidants and should be consumed regularly.
- If your diet is not ideal, supplement with I3C (400 mg/day) and rotate antioxidant supplements.

- Ground flaxseeds, one to two tablespoons per day, help metabolize estrogen more safely.
- Drink filtered water. (Use a filter that removes chlorine and heavy metals.)
- Eat organic, hormone-free meats and dairy.
- Choose paraben-free skin creams, makeup, and deodorant as much as possible.
- Store leftover foods in glass or ceramic. If wrapping cheese in plastic, cover it with parchment paper first. Oily foods absorb plastics more readily than other foods.
- Do not microwave foods in plastic containers or freeze water in plastic bottles.
- Drink green tea instead of coffee.
- Avoid fabric softeners or laundry detergents that use nonylphenol or octylphenol, which place petrochemicals in contact with your skin.
- Use natural forms of pest control.
- Avoid condoms with the spermicide nonoxyl-9, which breaks down into a xenoestrogen.

Know Your Symptoms

Let's talk about how you feel and what symptoms you are having, and the many reasons you may be feeling this way. As you will see, symptoms are key. They provide the clues to better understand your underlying imbalances. Most of us are looking for a quick fix, one pill to end our misery. The quick fixes are out there, in the form of Prozac and Ambien, to name just two, but if your mood is low or you're tossing and turning in the night, Prozac and Ambien won't fix the underlying problem. And these one-pill fixes don't usually last because the real problem has not been addressed. By getting rid of a symptom, you may feel better temporarily, but over time another symptom or two will emerge to make you miserable, either from a side effect of the very medication you've taken to feel better or from the actual root problem, which is being ignored.

I was watching television the other day when an antidepressant advertisement informed me that "seventy percent of all people taking antidepressants are still depressed." It went on to advise that if this is your problem, you should think about adding or switching to another antidepressant. Well, this can often work, but to me it confirmed what I see in my office: most medications work in the short term but eventually most people end up increasing their doses or adding more medications. Most prescription drugs act as a Band-Aid, to mask symptoms; they rarely treat the true, underlying problem. Sure, these medications have their place, but it is always better to "treat the root and not the leaf," as the ancient Chinese doctors used to say. If you are sleeping poorly, you need to explore what's wrong in your body and fix that rather than take a sleeping pill. If you lack energy, find the root cause, because you won't solve the problem with caffeine. In fact, you will probably only make matters worse, trading one symptom for another, such as insomnia or a stomach upset.

Everyone has symptoms of one sort or another, even the woman who thinks that "everything is just fine, thank you"—yes, even she has symptoms. Unfortunately we women have been groomed to accept our symptoms. We generally toe the party line and believe, as we've been told from our first menstrual pang, that our emotional ups and downs, bloats and belly pains are just part of being a girl. Menstruation has even been referred to as "the curse," and there are actually commercials on television advertising pills to limit the number of periods we must endure. Well, I would like to set the record straight. Symptoms are not part of being a girl. They are not to be ignored, medicated, denied, or even embraced. Symptoms need to be recognized and understood. They are the key to knowing your body is out of balance.

Menopause is not easy, but it can be easier to bear than peri-menopause, which is pretty much adolescence in reverse—and we all remember how unbearable adolescence was. In perimenopause, some nights you sleep and other nights you just don't. You often wake feeling sweaty and troubled. You can feel irritable and impatient and downright nasty. You no longer seem able to tolerate minor delays like slow-moving lines, automated answering systems, or incompetent people. Hairs start to sprout on your chin, wrinkles multiply and deepen, pubic hairs gray, and extra fat appears around your knees or waist despite the latest diet craze, step classes, or kickboxing. Sex can begin to feel like a chore and orgasms seem elusive or just not worth the effort. You feel too hot, or too sweaty, or too tired. Even the people you love can become a challenge. Perimenopause is not a great time to be dealing with teenagers, aging parents, lawyers, career changes, or haggling with siblings about whose turn it is to take Dad to the doctor. Let's face it, it can just plain suck. It is certainly not a time you want to embrace "the new you."

You may find yourself questioning what it is that really matters and what your priorities are. Forget about finding balance with work and family, you want balance for you. Menopause is all about you. Your life, your time.

The Chinese Perspective

I love the Chinese view of menopause. It helps to make sense of these changes. Chinese culture views a person's life in cycles. It recognizes cycles of seven. That is, every seven years there are major milestones, physically, physiologically, and spiritually. For example, at around age seven a greater sense of independence occurs, teeth fall out, molars crown, and kids want to understand more about why stuff happens. By age fourteen, menstruation has begun, hormones skyrocket, and emotions rage. At age twenty-one a person enters the world of work and starts making their dreams come true. Age twenty-eight marks a turning point so great that astrologers refer to it as the "Saturn return," when most people marry, divorce, or have children. And so it goes until the seventh cycle of seven, which the Chinese say is most important for women.

At this point, around age forty-nine, there is an actual shift in the way meridians flow in a woman's body. According to Chinese wisdom, a woman's innermost meridian (the conception vessel) closes, or becomes dry. With this, menstruation ceases and energy no longer flows outward from a woman's womb. Instead, we are told by the sages, energy rises upward toward the heart, and women become attuned to their innermost wisdom. Hence the term "wise old crone." So what does this mean for us menopausal women slugging it out in the modern world? I liken this process to a tsunami. Now, the last time a tsunami hit, there was an earthquake that measured 9.0 on the Richter scale, small islands were moved, and many people lost their lives. Menopause can feel like that.

Depending on your underlying physical and mental health, menopause can be tumultuous or calm. Chinese medicine recognizes that if a woman's yin energy is strong, she will have less trouble than if it is weak. That is, if there is strong yin to balance the yang, the body and the mind will be balanced. But if the yin is weak, then the yang energy rises, and hot flashes, headaches, and tempers will flare. There will be insomnia, breast pain, and spiritual upheaval—that is menopause as many of us know it.

So how do we gain better yin energy? The Chinese emphasize the kidney yin as being most deficient during menopause, and I liken kidney yin energy to adrenal function. These small glands overlying your kidneys are a powerhouse, designed to support your hormones as you age. You keep your adrenal glands working optimally by leading a balanced life—by getting proper rest, avoiding overeating and undereating, eating foods that are easy to digest and not overstimulating, getting proper exercise, and avoiding excess worry, anger, fear, grief, and even joy.

Now, if you are fortunate enough to have entered menopause with strong yin, then you are probably going to do well and thrive during menopause. But such good fortune is rare. The rest of us overworked, overstimulated, fast-food-fed baby boomers with aging parents and/or demanding kids and pets are going to have to work at it to get back on track. Here's how in a nutshell: you support your adrenal glands and the other glands they balance. Your symptoms and lab tests will help you determine which hormones are low and what you can do about it. When you are feeling more balanced, it will be easier to look at your lifestyle, which may be at the root of how you got out of balance in the first place.

Because hormones affect all organs, they affect all symptoms. I have found that treating hormonal imbalances can have the quickest and most dramatic impact on how you feel. When I see patients, I first balance their hormones. Not just one hormone, but all hormones that are too high or too low. I give my patients a hormone makeover and wait to see what symptoms are left.

Your Symptoms

I have found that for most women sleep, energy, and mood are the most important symptoms. Let's face it, no one likes any symptom, but if you are sleeping well and have good energy and a stable, positive mood, you can generally cope with most things. Sleep and energy are the more urgent symptoms to correct, because if you aren't sleeping through the night, your energy and mood will be off. If you lack energy, you aren't going to get things done in your life and you may feel discouraged. If your mood is low or changeable, you are going to have a hard time committing to any plan.

In addition to sleep, energy, and mood symptoms, you may have other symptoms such as headaches, unreliable bowels, anxiety, palpitations, and body aches. I call these minor symptoms. That is, they are usually not a major symptom of a hormone deficiency. Once a hormone or multiple hormones are brought back into balance, these symptoms generally improve. For example, you may have fatigue and find that your thyroid, though "normal," is not activating inside your cells. When you take a small dose of active thyroid (T3), you suddenly notice that not only does your energy improve but your hair stops falling out, your bowels become regular, and your skin and nails no longer crack.

Take this quiz to see what symptoms you may be having. Circle your answers to each question and then add up the numbers you've circled.

Signs/Symptoms	Never	Sometimes	Often/ Always
Major symptoms			
I have trouble sleeping.	0	5	10
I lack energy for what I need to do.	0	5	10
I am depressed.	0	5	10
I have mood swings/irritability.	0	5	10
Minor symptoms			
I feel tired, depressed, irritable with stress.	0	3	5
I have PMS symptoms.	0	3	5
I am not satisfied with my sex drive.	0	3	5
I have hot flashes.	0	3	5
I have headaches.	0	3	5
My hair is falling out.	0	2	4
My bowels are unreliable	0	2	4
I have anxiety.	0	2	4
I have palpitations.	0	2	4
I have body pains/aches.	0	2	4
I have started to look and feel old.	0	2	4

If you scored less than 10, you are doing pretty well. If you scored 10 to 20, you are just starting to need a hormonal tune-up. If you scored greater than 20, you definitely need some adjustments of your hormones. And if you scored over 30, read on, and begin your makeover now (or wither away, your choice).

How Hormones Affect Your Symptoms

There are many types of hormones, and they can help women of all ages, not just menopausal women with hot flashes. Most common minor symptoms such as dry skin, hair loss, joint pains, skin problems, and headaches are usually a sign of hormone imbalance. A hormone such as estrogen, for example, affects your energy, bowels, eyes, hair, and how your skin wrinkles. Many common complaints can improve with a blend of hormones. But it can be complicated—a particular symptom can be caused by more than one hormone problem, and usually more than one hormone is off. Your low energy could be caused by low thyroid hormone, low estrogen, low cortisol, low aldosterone, and/or low growth hormone. This can be confusing at first, but by looking closely at your symptoms and measuring hormone levels, you can figure out the likely cause of the problem and get back in balance.

Most of my patients complain of one or more of these five symptoms: insomnia, fatigue, low sex drive, mood problems, and looking older than they feel. These are also the symptoms that drive people to use sleeping pills or antidepressants or to seek plastic surgery. After you understand what hormones cause what symptoms (see appendixes A and B for a complete list), you can partner with your doctor to measure and support your hormones naturally. You will treat the root cause of your symptoms, and not only will your symptoms improve but you will also improve your long-term health.

The rest of this book will tell you what you need to know about using and monitoring hormones safely, as well as some things you can do to improve your own body's hormone production. Hormone support need not be for life, although it may be for some people. It should be used as needed to bring your body back into balance. With the right lifestyle, diet, and supplements, you may be able to reduce or stop hormonal supports. The important thing is to do what is right for you.

There's no one rule for everyone. We are all different. Our diets, stress levels, lifestyles, and genetics all vary, and they will continue to vary from year to year as we age. What is right for you at one time in your life may not be right at a later time.

Joan: Changing Hormone Supports through the Years

There is no magic pill that you can take for the rest of your life to stay healthy. As your body changes, your symptoms and treatment will have to change, too. Joan first came to see me when she was forty-two years old. She was stressed, overworked, and in a relationship that was full of drama. She was having terrible PMS symptoms every month. She'd had mild PMS symptoms in the past, but never so consistently and severely as now. In the six months before I met her, every month like clockwork, twelve days before her period, her mood and ability to cope would plummet and she was miserable. She would cry if a stranger looked at her crossly, and she noticed that her fingers became too fat for her rings and that her breasts were swollen and tender for days before her period. In addition, her bowels were sluggish for two weeks before her period, only to be loose when her bleeding began. She always felt better when her period started, and then the next month, it would all recur.

I recommended that she use vitex, an herb, to support her progesterone, in addition to vitamin B$_6$ and Chinese herbs. I also advised her to stop drinking so much caffeine and come for acupuncture treatments before her symptoms began each month. This worked magically, and within a month or two her PMS was vastly improved. (It is worth noting that as she improved, she came to recognize that her job was much too stressful and her boyfriend was a loser. She had never really understood that until her body came back into balance.) She changed jobs, ended her draining relationship, and began to feel so well that I did not hear from her other than for an annual Pap smear.

Six years later, at forty-eight, she reappeared in an anxious, distraught state. Her life had improved greatly. She had married a great guy and had a great job, but she had started to have "continuous PMS" with erratic heavy bleeding. She couldn't seem to fall asleep and she was depressed "for no reason." Sex was uncomfortable and unsatisfying. She had tried everything she knew, but the vitex and Chinese herbs were not helping anymore.

I explained that she was progressing through perimenopause, that her ovaries were aging and not responding to the herbs as they had in the past. We opted to use hormones instead of herbs. With a low dose of transdermal estradiol cream and progesterone capsules before bedtime on days 14 to 25 of her cycle, her symptoms improved greatly. The adrenal hormone DHEA was added with an adrenal extract and some liver herbs. Once again she regained her balance. We reviewed the symptoms of too much or too little of each of her hormones so she would know what symptoms to watch out for as her perimenopause progressed in the next year. As her body continues to age, I expect to see her again. Treatments have to change as we change.

Poor Sleep

"A good night's sleep is a treasure that all of the money in the world can't buy." I'm pretty sure that was written in the middle of the night by a wealthy perimenopausal insomniac. She recognized that without good sleep, life just isn't worth living. Difficulty sleeping is probably the most common symptom that I hear about from my female patients and the first problem that I try to correct. Without good sleep you cannot possibly expect to have good energy, a happy mood, or an exciting sex drive, or to look as good as you should.

Most of us sleep less than the recommended seven to eight hours per night, typically clocking in at a mere six hours nightly. Sleep surveys show that nearly half of the people in our country report some sleep problems, but from my experience it seems much higher, especially for women during perimenopause and menopause.

Many things affect our sleep, such as stress, foods, medications, temperature, sounds, and light. Even what we do before going to bed is important. Answering e-mails, watching TV shows about crime and murder, exercising, thinking about money and business, or planning the next day's agenda are all activities that are not conducive to sleep. Eating too late or drinking too much caffeine and/or alcohol are equally bad. Over-the-counter medications such as decongestants, pain pills, diet pills, cold/allergy medications, and sinus remedies often contain stimulants. Prescription medications, particularly antidepressants, asthma medications, blood pressure pills, and even sleeping pills (for prolonged periods), can cause or worsen insomnia.

Now, if you've considered these things, had your warm bath, "feng-shuied" your room, silenced your bed partner, and still can't sleep, consider your sex hormones.

- **Estrogen and progesterone** must be balanced for restful sleep. Often sleep problems are the very first sign of perimenopause. When I hear a thirty- or forty-something woman talk about her sleep issues, I think of progesterone first and foremost. **Progesterone** is sedating, calming, and relaxing. Just watch the slumber of a first-trimester pregnant woman—steeped in progesterone, she can literally sleep while standing. Ask a perimenopausal woman, who no longer makes enough progesterone, and she'll tell you that sleep is impossible, especially in the days just before her period. Just when you think things can't get much worse as you approach menopause, estrogen falls, in addition to progesterone, further interfering with your sleep—only now sleep is nearly impossible throughout your menstrual cycle. When this happens, and you lie awake in the dead of night with anxiety and maybe feeling too hot or too sweaty or both, you should consider estrogen. **Estrogen** enhances the production of serotonin and other neurotransmitters in our brain, which promote sleep, lift your mood, and enhance your sexual drive.
- The adrenal hormone **dehydroepiandrosterone (DHEA)** is our most abundant hormone. DHEA is also very important for sleep. It enhances our deepest phase of sleep and the REM (rapid eye movement) phase. During REM sleep you dream, and what is more important, you replenish the brain chemicals that control mood and create memories from the day's events. Without enough DHEA, your sleep will feel too light and you will not have many dreams. You may wake up feeling irritable. In addition to deepening sleep, DHEA boosts memory, mood, sex drive, and immune function, which are known to suffer from poor sleep.
- **Melatonin** is our major sleep hormone but it is also important for our long-term health. This ancient hibernation hormone is controlled by light, heat, and food, and it is often low during perimenopause. Without enough melatonin, your sleep is light.

You are easily awakened and once awake you find it hard to fall back to sleep. But melatonin is tricky. Too little, and you won't sleep well, but too much can also prevent restful sleep. Melatonin is also important for normal immunity, and without it you will age more quickly, have difficulty handling stress, and look haggard and older than your years.

- **Thyroid hormone** is not normally recognized as being important for sleep, but without enough thyroid hormone, your sleep will not feel refreshing and may even be uncomfortable due to aches and muscle cramps. Thyroid hormone levels can be normal according to routine thyroid blood tests, but inside your cells, thyroid hormone may not be activated. Though your blood tests look fine, your cells and you feel otherwise. There are many reasons that you could have problems activating thyroid hormone, such as low adrenal hormones (particularly DHEA) or low minerals such as magnesium, iodine, selenium, or iron. Many medications can interfere with thyroid activation, such as birth control pills, beta-blockers, and nonsteroidal anti-inflammatory drugs. We may feel that this is happening, but often the only way to know for sure is with a twenty-four-hour urine test to measure the T3 inside the cells (discussed in chapters 6 and 10).

- **Cortisol** levels should also be followed. Cortisol is our major stress hormone and gives us stamina. It keeps our body ready to fight foes, battle infections, and balance our sugar. It is produced in a cyclic fashion according to our natural circadian rhythm, and this rhythm is vital for a good night's sleep. A high evening or night-time level of cortisol will make falling or staying asleep impossible. The problem is not that we have too much cortisol, as most television commercials would have you believe, it is rather that our cortisol regulation is poor. Cortisol should normally be high first thing in the morning and gradually fall as the day wears on. Many people with weak adrenal glands lose their cortisol rhythm, with low daytime cortisols and high evening or early-morning cortisol levels. This is one of the most common causes of sleep disturbance that I see, and it will only be discovered by checking cortisol levels throughout the day and night (easily done with a saliva test). Phosphatidylserine (100 to 500 mg/day) is a supplement that helps to stabilize cortisol and can improve this problem. As people age, their cortisol rhythm tends to become more and more disrupted, giving rise to the early-morning waking often seen in the elderly.

- **Growth hormone** is primarily made when you are most deeply asleep. This can be a problem for insomniacs and shift workers. Growth hormone gives restful and refreshing sleep. The depth of sleep seen in babies and young children, who have the highest growth hormone levels of all humans, is a testament to its sleep-enhancing effects. There is much debate about using growth hormone, but it has been a mainstay of the anti-aging community for over twenty years. Improving low growth hormone levels, by using either injections or amino acid–based growth hormone "enhancers" can dramatically improve your sleep if your growth hormone is too low.

Hormonal Causes and Characteristics of Poor Sleep

Estrogen   Sleep that is too light, waking unrefreshed even if sleeping through the night.

Progesterone   PMS insomnia, trouble falling asleep, difficulty falling back if awakened.

DHEA   Sleep that feels too light, lacking dreams.

Melatonin   Difficulty falling asleep, awakening in the night suddenly anxious, fewer dreams.

Cortisol   Difficulty falling asleep or early waking (if cortisol level is too high in the evening or early morning, say 4 to 5 a.m.). Waking unrefreshed despite sleeping through the night (if cortisol is deficient in the morning).

Thyroid   Waking unrefreshed with puffy lids, muscle aches, tendency to snore; waking frequently.

Growth Hormone   Need for more than nine hours of sleep to get any rest, wake feeling exhausted; sleep is light and unrefreshing even if sleeping throughout the night.

Low Energy

Being tired a lot is not normal, but it is very common. Studies show that not having enough energy to do what you want to do is one of the top ten reasons that people go to a doctor. Unless the cause is organic, such as an underlying illness, infection, poor diet, or anemia, many leave their doctor's office no more enlightened or energized. Yet fatigue is one of the most frequent and easiest symptoms that I routinely treat.

Most symptoms of fatigue improve once you are sleeping well and your hormones are balanced. There are many reasons for hormone imbalance, such as deficiency of minerals (particularly magnesium); overwork; lack of sleep or exercise; excess travel; unrelenting stress; poor diet; and aging itself. Remember, we are all destined to experience a gradual decline in hormones by our early forties, and how you fare depends very much on your life circumstances (stress, illness, accidents) and how well you nourish yourself (diet, exercise, rest). So if you are feeling tired, know that hormones can help.

In general, hormonally caused fatigue improves quickly, within hours or days after starting support. The trick is using the right amount of energizing hormones so that sleep is not adversely affected. There may be clues as to which hormone is low depending on when your fatigue is worst. For example, fatigue that is worse in the early morning, making it hard to get out of bed, is often a sign of low thyroid hormone. Fatigue that worsens as the day goes on—the "3 p.m. blues"—may be a sign of low adrenal hormones, particularly cortisol. Fatigue that lasts all day long is often due to a lack of estradiol, and fatigue that is worse if you stay out too late or have too much fun, despite adequate sleep—"payback fatigue"—may be a sign of low growth hormone. Fatigue that is worse after being on your feet too long signals a problem with aldosterone; a general lack of endurance could be from other low adrenal hormones, DHEA, pregnenolone, and/or epinephrine.

Hormonal Causes of Low Energy

Estradiol   Constant tiredness, tired out by regular activities.

Cortisol   Fatigue worse in the afternoon (3 to 4 p.m.), fatigue worsened by stress or exercise, improved with rest.

DHEA   Lack of endurance for daily activities.

Pregnenolone   Low endurance, lack of energy and enthusiasm for regular activities.

Aldosterone   Lack of endurance, worse if upright, also sleepy when seated upright (during lectures, or movies, for example).

Thyroid   Worse with rest and in the morning, hard to wake up or get started for the day.

Growth Hormone   Payback fatigue, if you exert yourself or stay out too late.

Mood Problems

Depression affects some 20 million Americans, and most depressed Americans are women, perimenopausal or menopausal. We have become a nation with a high population of medicated and sedated women. That is not to say that we haven't greatly improved upon medieval treatments for depression, which included torture and drowning to rid the soul of demons, but I think we can do better.

At the turn of the twentieth century, Freud suggested that someday an organic cause would be found to explain depression. Then modern science discovered the role that neurotransmitters such as serotonin, dopamine, and norepinephrine play. Only recently have we begun to understand how neurotransmitters are affected by our hormones.

Estrogen, a very yang hormone, acts to raise serotonin levels, elevating our mood, improving our memory, and greatly enhancing our sex drive. We naturally have a calming yin hormone, progesterone, to balance estrogen's yang. Progesterone prevents hysteria and calms our moods, largely by raising levels of neurotransmitters such as GABA (gamma-aminobutyric acid) and dopamine. GABA is a calming neurotransmitter, a bit like Valium, which reduces anxiety and induces sleep. Dopamine also supports sex drive and curbs our appetite. When these hormones are out of balance, you've got an angry, carbohydrate-craving woman who can't sleep.

Antidepressants have been the most popular answer to menopausal symptoms. They will help to raise your mood, but your sex drive, sexy curves, bones, memory, skin, and even your heart health may take a dive. Antidepressants have their place, but they cannot and should not replace your natural hormones to improve your mood.

The adrenal hormones cortisol and DHEA are powerful mood elevators and are often out of balance in perimenopause and beyond. These hormones, which support our kidney yin, support all of our hormones as we age. Without enough cortisol, we lack enthusiasm and energy. Without enough DHEA, our sex drive and mood are flat. That being said, you might be surprised to learn that many depressed people have high cortisol levels. As I just explained in the previous section, high levels of cortisol do not necessarily mean that there is too much cortisol. It usually implies that the cortisol control is poor and the normal circadian rhythm is lost. Cortisol may be high in the late afternoon or evening, when it should be winding down. Over time, as cortisol becomes more depleted, feelings of depression worsen. I have read reports and even hear on TV commercials that women have too much cortisol. But I have been measuring twenty-four-hour levels in women for years and I can attest that this is rarely the case. Rather, women typically have low, or low normal, amounts of cortisol and other adrenal hormones, with poor control of their cortisol rhythm, resulting in high levels of cortisol in the afternoon that cause afternoon binge eating and insomnia. Many of us double-tasking, working women have worn-out adrenal glands. Often we can rally through, but when we hit perimenopause and our ovaries wind down, adrenal symptoms can appear as depression. Rest, meditation, yoga, good food, and lots of sleep can help, but if you can't afford a health spa (and even if you can), support your adrenal glands. Most women improve dramatically with some adrenal supports, such as adrenal extracts, cortisol, or herbs. As your adrenal glands recover, they will regain their natural rhythm and can even help make more sex hormones. Your cortisol rhythm is restored and your feelings of anxiety and irritability will improve; you'll sleep more soundly and have a better mood, naturally.

Growth hormone helps you deal with stress. I like to think of it as the problem-solving hormone. When growth hormone levels are low, one tends to feel victimized or easily overwhelmed by day-to-day problems—the "Why me?" complex. When growth hormone levels are restored, these daily problems don't seem like such a big deal, just something to fix. Anxiety levels fall, and you can see the bigger picture.

Melatonin is not traditionally thought of as a hormone that affects mood, but it does. When melatonin levels are low, you tend to wake in the wee hours in a panicked state, even if things may be generally okay in your life. You will wake fearing the worst about the least important things or feeling depressed for no real reason. Melatonin is made from the amino acid tryptophan, which also makes serotonin. Its production in the brain requires methionine and SAMe (S Adenosyl methionine).

SAMe has been prescribed for years in Europe to treat depression, and recently it became available in the United States without a prescription. It is particularly helpful in treating depression, particularly depression with fatigue, as it can be very energizing. For this reason I always start SAMe at low doses (say, 100 to 200 mg in the morning) and increase it gradually. It should be used with a health practitioner's advice, as it can cause anxiety and insomnia if the dose is too high.

Thyroid hormones are essential for normal mood, and thyroid hormone deficiency is a well-known cause of depression. When thyroid hormones are too low, the mood is typically lowest first thing in the morning. You wake with a sense of dread for the coming day. Symptoms are usually better as you get going but may worsen if you rest for a prolonged period, or nap. Excess thyroid hormones can cause anxiety or panic attacks.

Hormone Deficiencies Affecting How You Feel

Estrogen   Depression worse during or just after the menstrual period or with menopause.

Progesterone   Anxiety/irritability in the week or two before the menstrual period.

Cortisol   Anxiety/irritability worse late in the day or worse with stress.

Thyroid   Depression worse when first waking in the morning or when resting or napping.

DHEA   Nervous, irritable, anxious, with a low sex drive.

Aldosterone   Mood is worse if on your feet all day and better when you rest lying flat.

Melatonin   Nighttime anxiety, depression in the middle of the night.

Growth Hormone   Lack of self-confidence, feeling victimized by problems ("Why me?"), vulnerable to stress, easily discouraged.

Looking Older Than You Should

We live in a country with a $15 billion obsession with good looks. Plastic surgery, lasers, skin peels, liposuction, and Botox injections may make you look better, but they won't prevent further signs or symptoms of aging, not to mention their expense and possible side effects. Plastic surgery is much like a new coat of paint on an old car. Wrinkles, sagging skin, hair loss, facial hair, and weight gain are usually caused by hormonal imbalance and deficiency. Supporting your hormones will not only make you feel better than any plastic surgery, it can enhance the procedures you may be destined to try. When I attend anti-aging conferences, roughly half of the audience are plastic surgeons, who know that without hormone support their handiwork is doomed to deteriorate all too quickly.

- **Progesterone** is usually the first hormone to decline in women. As progesterone levels fall, breasts tend to swell and become tender. Women often complain that their bra size and weight increase during perimenopause. Low progesterone can also cause your ankles and fingers to swell and your stomach to bloat.
- **Estrogen deficiency**, the hallmark of menopause, first shows up in a woman's face, somewhere in her thirties and forties. Fine lines begin to etch her forehead, the corners of her eyes, and around her mouth, fondly called "smile lines," or worse, "crow's feet" or "worry lines." As your estrogen begins to fall (some ten years before you hit menopause), hair often thins on your scalp but starts to grow on your face. Breasts shrivel and sag.
- **Thyroid hormone deficiency** causes a host of aging signs such as thinning eyebrows, brittle or splitting nails, thinning hair, and dry skin. Weight gain is common and there may be swelling of the lower legs. Low thyroid function causes problems metabolizing cholesterol and beta-carotene, resulting in low vitamin A and high beta-carotene levels. This manifests in subtle signs, like yellowed or slightly sallow skin color (high beta-carotene), goose bumps on the backs of the upper arms, and deeply calloused heels (low vitamin A). Vitamin A is toxic in high doses for prolonged periods of time (it can cause liver failure and vaginitis) but it can be used safely with the guidance of a doctor to alleviate skin problems and even reduce heavy bleeding (it improves mucous membranes such as the uterine lining and the cervix).
- **Growth hormone deficiency** is a plastic surgeon's dream. It causes droopy eyelids and sagging cheeks. Wrinkles deepen and a deep

groove is seen in the cheeks as the skin loses its elasticity. The muscles, particularly the triceps in the back of the arms, become flaccid and hang. The upper lip begins to thin and the jawline becomes less prominent. Weight gain is typical, with an increase in cellulite production and sagging fat at the knees. The skin tends to dehydrate with fine wrinkles, unkindly referred to as "elephant skin."

- **Low cortisol** gives rise to skin rashes and inflammations of any kind, which shouldn't come as too much of a surprise. What do you put on inflamed skin? Topical cortisone. Joints and skin inflame when cortisol is too low. The eyelids tend to redden and the face can have an unhealthy ruddy appearance. Eczema, seborrheic dermatitis, hives, vitiligo, and pigmentations often occur, and brown age spots can appear on the face and lower arms. Look at the eyes of most eighty-year-olds and you will see the inflamed eyelids so characteristic of low cortisol.

- **Inadequate DHEA** gives rise to a tendency toward a flabby belly and increased production of cellulite, particularly in the thighs. The eyes become dry and lusterless, and the skin and hair lose their glow due to a lack of natural oils.

- **Low melatonin** causes you to look older than you really are, and you may even gray prematurely. People with low melatonin often appear tired and have anxious-looking eyes. They look like they have slept poorly, and this is probably so.

Low Hormones Affect How You Look

Estrogen   Bone loss, wrinkles around mouth/eyes/forehead, increasing facial hair, dry eyes, thinning scalp hair.

Thyroid   Thinning eyebrows/hair, gooseflesh on upper arms, dry skin with swelling, cold hands and feet with skin peeling around the cuticles, skin may be yellowish, thinning hair.

DHEA   Face dull/lacking luster, skin and hair are dry, less body or pubic hair, thinned underarm hair.

Cortisol   Reddened eyelids/cheeks, eczema, hives, rashes.

Growth Hormone   Deepened wrinkles in the face, thinned upper lip, receding jaw.

Melatonin   Tired, anxious face; premature aging.

Low Sex Drive

The typical orgasm lasts twelve seconds in both men and women, and averages about twelve minutes in total per year. Yet it consumes a great deal of our waking thoughts. Women like sex every bit as much as men, and we miss it as we age. Let's face it, with age, orgasms can become more elusive or less intense. Research has clearly shown that sex drive decreases with age in both men and women, and this decline begins in the fourth or fifth decade, coinciding with a decline in sex hormones.

Sexual function is often the last symptom to improve and can be the most resistant to treatment. There are, of course, many reasons for this. Antidepressants, overwork, stress, insomnia, marital strain, life, worry, and a low mood will dampen any sexual stirrings. In menopause, women's stress levels are often highest, compared with any other age. Our bodies change as well. The vaginal lining becomes thinner, less flexible, and less moist, and for this reason urinary and vaginal infections are common. Your G-spot in the PC (pubococcygeal) muscle, the most common source of orgasm in women, may require greater stimulation to "ring the bell."

We are inundated by commercials promising improved sexual function for men, but what these commercials fail to mention is that although erectile dysfunction will improve with Viagra and the like, passion will not. Passion, that joie de vivre feeling that dwindles with age in both men and women, is often a symptom of low hormones. Hormones definitely improve sex, and this is particularly true for estradiol (for women) and testosterone (for men). As important as sex hormones are, without adequate thyroid, cortisol, and growth hormone, sex drive will not be fully restored. In addition, the adrenal hormone DHEA plays an important role for both sexes in enhancing feelings of sexual desire. As you can see, it typically takes several hormones for sex to be easy and fun from midlife onward.

The Next Step

Perhaps you're feeling a bit overwhelmed with all these hormones. But take it one step at a time. The next step should be to measure your hormone levels and then find the right sort of support to bring back hormone balance. By now you may already suspect what hormones need to be checked in you. Chapter 6 will help you figure out what tests to take. And then we'll talk about how to find the right doctor. You can't do this alone.

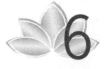

Recommended Tests

There is an ongoing debate about the best tests to measure each hormone. In fact, there is even debate among physicians as to what is a true "normal" value for certain hormones. Why? Because hormones change throughout the day and night, and they are constantly changing depending on your age, diet, stress levels, genetics, physical activity, and body size. What is a normal level for a sedentary eighty-year-old, ninety-pound woman is definitely not going to be normal for an active, forty-year-old, two-hundred-pound man. Yet ranges of "normal" thyroid values for most labs are the same for both! To complicate matters further, hormones can be measured from the blood, urine, or saliva.

In most cases, actual hormone levels don't matter as much as how you feel, but knowing hormone levels can be helpful for a few reasons: (1) if you are uncertain which hormone is causing a certain symptom; (2) to ensure your hormone dose is adequate and that you are absorbing enough hormone from a hormone cream or lotion; (3) to ensure that your hormone dose is not too high; and (4) to see if your hormones are breaking down (metabolizing) safely in your body. The best way to measure hormones depends on many things, such as which hormone is being measured, costs of tests, insurance coverage, and availability of testing.

Measuring Hormones

It's important to understand a few things about how your hormones work and what tests are available in order to get the right test: (1) There are binding proteins in your body that can prevent hormones from doing their job. These proteins have to be considered when interpreting test results. (2) The timing of the measurements is important because some of our hormones peak at certain times of the day. (3) The wrong test (blood, urine, or saliva) may not give you all the information you need. (4) Normal values are not always valid. (5) You need to consider costs. Some insurance plans will only cover tests from specific labs; other plans cover outside specialty labs. If you have no insurance, or limited funds, urine or saliva testing may be the most informative and cost-effective.

Free and Bound Hormones

Hormones are powerful. They affect your brain, bones, liver, breasts, bowels, muscles—essentially every cell in your body. They don't just float around in your bloodstream freely, they are attached to binding proteins (albumin, or binding globulins) that carry them to various parts of your body safely. You could think of this like a limousine service. The limo picks up free hormones, usually in the liver, and delivers them to their final destination, usually at a cell receptor, somewhere in the body.

Hormones that are being carried by binding proteins are not free to act in the body, as they are "bound." They can act only when they get out of the limo and are free (which happens at the final destination, or cell receptor). Your body could actually have normal amounts of hormones in it, but if most of those hormones are bound to binding globulins or other proteins, your hormones aren't free to act and you will have all of the signs and symptoms of a hormone deficiency, despite normal blood levels. For this reason when you measure hormones, particularly thyroid hormone and testosterone, a free level must be checked. Urine and saliva tests only measure free hormones. Blood tests may measure free levels, but this is not always done and must be specifically requested.

Sex Hormone Binding Globulin

Sex hormone binding globulin (SHBG) is the main protein (the limo) that carries sex hormones (estrogen, progesterone, and testosterone) around in your body, but it can also pick up thyroid hormone and cortisol. Because SHBG levels rise as we age, they bind more hormones and our free hormone levels fall. Because hormones are naturally falling as we grow older, an increasing SHBG only worsens our hormone deficiencies. We feel more and more hormonally deprived. Another problem with SHBG is that it can change cells so that they don't respond as well to other hormones, such as insulin. This is a reason that older people are more prone to adult-onset diabetes.

SHBG is made in the liver. When sex hormones are taken orally (by mouth), they are absorbed in the gut and pass directly into the liver. The liver is not used to seeing high levels of hormones, so it responds by making extra SHBG to bind them. Over time, when using oral hormones (including birth control pills and oral estrogen), SHBG levels will rise, often to double the normal level. High SHBG proteins bind not only our estrogen, but testosterone, cortisol, and thyroid hormones. This explains why women taking oral hormones over time often complain of lower sex drive, vaginal dryness, and fatigue, or they start to feel as if their hormones are just not as strong as they used to be. If you are taking estrogen by mouth, it is important to measure your SHBG to learn if it is interfering with your hormones. Better yet, switch to a hormone skin cream or lotion. Because the hormones are absorbed through your skin, they bypass your liver and don't cause a high rise in SHBG.

Timing of Tests

Your body makes some hormones at certain times of day only; some hormone production even depends on your activities. Cortisol peaks in the morning. Thyroid hormones become more active when you are more active. Melatonin and growth hormones peak in the middle of the night. Estrogen varies with your menstrual cycle, highest from mid-cycle onward and lowest during menstruation. Progesterone production usually peaks around day 20 of the menstrual cycle and falls abruptly about a week later, bringing on your period. Aldosterone levels are lowest when you are at rest and lying down, and they rise when you are active and standing or sitting upright. For these reasons, simple blood tests are not always the best way to see how well your hormones are doing. They are like a snapshot that may have been taken at the wrong time to get the full picture.

On the other hand, twenty-four-hour urine tests measure free hormone levels throughout the day. This can be very helpful if you feel that a hormone level is low but blood tests insist that you are normal. Saliva tests for cortisol, measured at various times throughout the day, can explain why you feel tired or are overeating in the late afternoon, or why you have trouble falling asleep in the evening or wake up in the middle of the night. In general, if you measure a hormone to see if it is too low, check it when the level should be highest. At this point it should be in the mid- to upper-middle-range of normal. If you are trying to determine if a hormone is too high or is being absorbed from your skin cream, measure it between doses.

Which Test Is Best?

Blood, urine, and saliva testing all have their place among the tools you need to measure your hormones. Measuring hormones can be confusing because there are so many ways to do it. Certainly, blood testing is the most common and widely accepted method of measuring hormone levels. However, as you've seen, it is not always the most reliable or the most cost-effective. You don't want to waste money on a test that won't give you the information you need. Here are some basic rules to help you decide which test is best:

- It isn't always necessary to test. In menopause it isn't necessary to measure estrogen levels if you are obviously low as indicated by your symptoms (for example, hot flashes and/or night sweats). Progesterone also doesn't need to be measured in menopause, as it is only produced when you are having menstrual cycles. However, once you are on hormone support, blood or urine hormone tests are important to ensure that you are absorbing hormones adequately and that the dose is ideal.
- Twenty-four-hour urine tests measure metabolites, which are important to ensure that your body is breaking down your hormones in a safe way. This is especially important for DHEA and estrogen.
- Saliva testing when using transdermal hormones is not reliable. Hormones applied to the skin concentrate in the saliva and contamination from the skin usually causes hormone levels to be very high. Levels in the saliva are reported as too high, even though the body dose is normal. More labs are now providing salivary ranges but I generally do not use saliva levels except for measuring cortisol, melatonin, and DHEA.
- Sex hormones vary throughout the menstrual cycle. If you are still menstruating, progesterone is best measured on days 19 to 21, when it peaks. Because estrogen levels are more variable, the best time to measure estrogen levels is when you have symptoms such as headache, low mood, or low energy, or during the week of the cycle when production is at its all-time low. If estradiol levels are falling below 60 pg/ml, estrogen support most likely will improve many symptoms.

In a perfect world—that is, if there are no financial or insurance barriers to testing—when I first meet a patient, I routinely order the following blood and urine tests, which are ideally done before any hormone therapies are started to serve as a baseline, obtained first thing in the morning:

Blood Tests

- Thyroid: TSH, free T3, free T4 (free tests must be requested, as they are not part of a routine thyroid panel) and antithyroid antibodies (the most common cause of thyroid disease in women in this country).
- Testosterone levels, both free and total.

- Adrenal hormones: Cortisol (the morning level is preferable, as this is when it peaks), DHEA-S, aldosterone, and pregnenolone.
- Vitamin D (25-hydroxy vitamin D): If it's too low, you are at increased risk of bone loss (less than 30 ng/ml, although many sources recommend levels above 50 ng/ml).
- Homocysteine: Measures how well your body is methylating. If levels are too high, you are at risk for heart disease and may have difficulty breaking down your estrogen. Some physicians recommend taking 1000 to 1500 mg methionine six hours before the blood test, because homocystiene levels may be (falsely) low if you are deficient in methionine.
- Tests for minerals are important for hormone function, particularly iron and magnesium. Magnesium is the most common mineral deficiency in adults. You must request an RBC (red blood cell) magnesium level, as regular serum levels don't measure the level inside your cells, where it matters. A ferritin level measures your iron stores, which influence thyroid performance.
- CBC (complete blood count).
- Chemistry panel: Measures liver function, calcium, albumin, and body salts affected by adrenal hormones.
- If you are cycling, estradiol level should be checked on the day of symptoms or during the week of menstruation, when estrogen levels are lowest. Progesterone should be measured when it is normally peaking, days 19 to 21 of your cycle. If cycles are irregular, FSH and LH should be measured to see if menopause is the cause. If you are not having cycles, prolactin levels should be measured to make sure your pituitary gland is working normally. In menopause, if you are on estrogen and progesterone support, measure blood levels only to ensure that your hormone levels are adequate and safe.

Urine tests are very useful. Twenty-four-hour urine collections can be tedious, but they measure hormone breakdown (metabolites) and can measure hormones that normally fluctuate throughout the day. I like to obtain them on my patients to get a baseline and as a follow-up once each year.

Urine tests

- Twenty-four-hour urine tests measure estrogen metabolites, progesterone metabolites, DHEA and its metabolites, DHT, cortisol, aldosterone, free T3, and growth hormone.
- Morning urine tests are available to measure epinephrine, norepinephrine, serotonin, and dopamine. These tests are typically done in the morning two hours after waking up, when these neurotransmitters are peaking.
- First-morning urine tests can measure growth hormone and some labs are starting to offer melatonin metabolites from them as well.

Saliva tests

- Saliva testing is a great way to follow cortisol throughout the day and night. Morning saliva can measure DHEA, and nighttime tests measure melatonin.

Specialty Labs

ALCAT Worldwide
1239 E. Newport Center Drive, Suite 101
Deerfield Beach, FL 33442
Phone: 800-872-5228
www.alcat.com

ALCAT Worldwide offers testing for food allergies and toxic exposures.

Doctor's Data Inc.
3755 Illinois Avenue
St. Charles, IL 60174
Phone: 630-377-8139
www.doctorsdata.com

Doctor's Data Inc. offers heavy metal testing, red cell mineral assessments, and digestive analysis.

Genova Diagnostics
63 Zillicoa Street
Asheville, NC 28801
Phone: 800–522–4762
www.GDX.net

Genova Diagnostics provides genetic "SNPs" to assess which enzyme pathways you may have inherited that could predispose you to heart disease, cancer, or clotting. It provides twenty-four-hour urine tests for all hormones and hormone metabolites, as well as blood levels for many antioxidants and vitamins. It also offers digestive analysis in addition to stool tests for glucuronidase, detox, and metabolic profiles, as well as organic acid tests.

The Great Plains Laboratory, Inc.
11813 W. 77th Street
Lenexa, KS 66214
Phone: 913-341-8949
Fax: 913-341-6207
www.greatplainslaboratory.com

The Great Plains Laboratory, Inc. offers a metabolic test known as Organic Acids that can provide a picture of how well your detox systems are working (glutathione and vitamin C levels), vitamin levels (particularly B vitamins), and how well your digestion is working

Igenex Labs
795 San Antonio Road
Palo Alto, CA 94303
Phone: 800-832-3200
www.igenex.com

Igenex Labs offers testing for Lyme and other tick-borne diseases. I do such testing in patients whose adrenal or immune function is not improving as I would expect.

NeuroScience
373 280th Street
Osceola, WI 54020
Phone: 715-755-3995
www.neurorelief.com

NeuroScience performs tests on urinary neurotransmitter levels as well as saliva testing for cortisol, DHEA, and melatonin. They offer targeted amino acid therapies to treat symptoms of anxiety, insomnia, and depression.

Quest Diagnostics (and the regular lab your doctor uses)

Quest Diagnostics labs are located throughout the country and many doctors use them routinely. They can perform many of the routine blood tests mentioned throughout this book, such as RBC magnesium, homocysteine, CRP, DHEA-S, all hormone levels, SHBG, and IGF-1. They also offer specialized tests such as CoQ10 levels and vitamin A and vitamin E levels, so be sure to ask your doctor if he or she uses Quest or a comparable lab.

Rhein Consulting Laboratories
4475 SW Scholls Ferry Road, Suite 101
Portland, OR 97225
Phone: 503-292-1988
www.rheinlabs.com

Rhein Consulting Laboratories does excellent and affordable twenty-four-hour urine tests for all hormone metabolites. They plan to offer urinary growth hormone levels in the future.

Spectracell Laboratories
10401 Town Park Drive
Houston, Texas 77072
713-621-3101
www.spectracell.com

Spectracell Laboratories provides comprehensive blood analysis to measure antioxidants, vitamins, and lipids (fats) important for heart health.

How to Find the Right Doctor and Support Team

Finding the right doctor is key to maintaining your health. In today's world many of us find ourselves in a managed care setting with what can sometimes feel like too few options. Some health insurance companies dictate your care by assigning you a doctor, which is a bit like an arranged marriage: sometimes it works out, sometimes not. Sadly, many patients complain to me that "I don't really like my doctor," or that "My doctor hardly knows me," or worse, "My doctor seems uninterested in me." Their complaints are too often well founded. We live in a fast-paced world, and many doctors see patients for only about fifteen to thirty minutes, hardly enough time to discuss sleep, mood, weight, energy, and life-cycle changes as intricate and confusing as peri-menopause and beyond. If you have no one you trust or not enough time to discuss options, you can easily feel overwhelmed and abandoned. To make matters worse, we are bombarded by advertisements for sleep aids, mood elevators, and vaginal lubricants, in addition to the conflicting media reports of scary studies warning of dangers in the very cures we seek. Doctors get bombarded with all of this hoopla, too, and sometimes become just as misinformed as everyone else. What do you do? Take charge. Seek good, reliable partners for your health. They are out there.

I need to digress here to say something about the way many of us approach health care. Most of us treat our cars better than our bodies. We all have car insurance to cover us in the event of an accident, and we understand that we also have a deductible, a sum of money that we have to pay before our insurance kicks in. Certainly we don't expect our car insurance to cover the cost of new tires, oil changes, and other routine maintenance. And when our car is making loud, scary noises, we don't ignore it. We take it to a good mechanic. Not just any mechanic; we find someone we can trust. We need to learn to view our health in this same way. Insurance companies cannot do it all for us, and life is about choices. Most health insurance is typically great for catastrophes and hospitalizations but not so great for our day-to-day maintenance. That's where you need to take charge and decide what your priorities are and what you can do for yourself. You need to seek out a practitioner whom you like and trust, someone who will take the time to listen and get to know you, a true partner. Be proactive with your health care. You may need to pay for some specialty testing or expert consulting on your own. Generally you should only need to use specialty labs once or twice a year to measure metabolites or check neurotransmitter levels. These are often covered by insurance, but if not, don't let that be a barrier to your good health. Think of it like car maintenance.

If you don't like your doctor, or your doctor is not spending enough time getting to know you, or not really listening or treating you the way you want, then change. Make it a priority and do some research. Talk to other women. Ask compounding pharmacists; call specialty labs. When you get a name, do more research. Call to see if the office is helpful and organized. Ask about treatments. Does the doctor offer natural hormone treatments? How long is a typical new-patient visit and follow-up visit? Once you're an established patient, is there a long wait to get in for an emergency? Does the doctor have any special interests or training? More and more physicians are learning to think outside the box. They understand that truly preventive medicine doesn't mean simply diagnosing disease earlier, it is about disease prevention. There are many organizations listed at the end of this chapter where doctors train in natural medicine. Call them for a doctor in your area.

How to Find a Compounding Pharmacy

The world of natural hormones came alive for me when I was introduced to the world of compounding pharmacists. A compounding pharmacist is a pharmacist trained to prepare medications in all forms: oral (by mouth), transdermal (via the skin), sublingual (under the tongue), or by injection. Compounding is not a new concept. In the past all pharmacists regularly compounded medications. Compounding pharmacists can provide medications and hormone preparations that are free of the problems associated with standard medical prescriptions. That is, they create individualized prescriptions in any dose, measuring out precise doses on request. These pharmacists are like the pharmacists of years ago. They can make any cream or lotion from any base and make a hormone preparation as strong or weak as you need. They can put vitamins and antioxidants into tablets, or they can simply help you with dosing or with questions about using natural hormones. Compounding pharmacists are located in every state, and you can find one near you by going online to the International Academy of Compounding Pharmacists' Web site (www.iacprx.org). A compounding pharmacist in your area may also be able to tell you which physicians near you are using natural hormones and where to go for saliva, blood, and urine testing.

Compounded hormones have been criticized recently for not having FDA approval. This is a misleading criticism. Because compounded medications are produced for an individual patient as prescribed by a physician, they are not regulated by the FDA. They are not a single drug, but vary from prescription to prescription. Compounded medications are regulated by individual state boards of pharmacy, not by the FDA. The pharmacist works in conjunction with a prescribing physician to meet the needs of you, the patient, individually. If we learned one thing from the WHI study, it is that women cannot all be given the same pill, the same dose, without first considering who they are as individuals. Compounding pharmacies can do this.

How do you know if what you get from the compounding pharmacy is good? Most compounding pharmacies routinely have their products tested by an independent source to ensure that the concentration of their products contains the prescribed dose. You should ask your pharmacist or prescribing doctor if this is done routinely, particularly if you do not feel a treatment is working as expected.

The Next Step

Once you've determined your symptoms and/or measured your hormone levels with a doctor you trust, the next step is to bring your hormone levels back into balance. Always tackle your biggest problems first. Getting a good night's sleep, enough energy for your day, and a stable mood should take priority. Starting with the sex hormones, estrogen and progesterone, is the best way to begin.

Compounding Pharmacies

Bird's Hill Pharmacy
401 Great Plain Avenue
Needham, MA 02492
781-449-0550 or 888-500-2660
www.birdshill.com

College Pharmacy
3505 Austin Bluff Parkway
Suite 101
Colorado Springs, CO 80918
800-888-9358
www.collegepharmacy.com

International Academy of Compounding Pharmacists
P.O. Box 1365
Sugarland, TX 77487
800-927-4227 (toll-free referral line)
Iacpinfo@iacprx.org
www.iacprx.org

Pierce Apothecary
1180 Beacon Street
Brookline, MA 02446
617-566-4080
www.jepierce.com

University Compounding Pharmacy
1875 Third Avenue
San Diego, CA 92101
866-444-9475 or 800-985-8065
www.ucprx.com

Women's International Pharmacy
12012 N. 111th Avenue
Youngtown, AZ 85363
800-279-5708
www.womensinternational.com

Doctors Who Use
Natural Hormones

American Academy of Anti-Aging Medicine
1510 W. Montana Street
Chicago, Il 60614
773-528-6100
www.worldhealth.net

American Academy of Medical Acupuncture
www.medicalacupuncture.org

American Association of Naturopathic Physicians
4435 Wisconsin Avenue
Washington, D.C. 20016
202-237-8150
www.naturopathic.org

American College for Advancement in Medicine
24411 Ridge Route
Suite 115
Laguna Hills, CA 92653
949-309-3520
www.acam.org

American Holistic Medical Association
P.O. Box 2016
Edmonds, WA 98020
425-967-0737
www.holisticmedicine.org

Institute for Functional Medicine
www.functionalmedicine.org

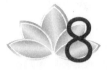

Sex Hormones Part 1: Perimenopause and Progesterone

Women's sex hormones, estrogen and progesterone (with a little help from testosterone), pretty much run the world. Biologically our main purpose is to survive and procreate. Pregnancy, one of our most important responsibilities, is a miraculous, mysterious series of events controlled and fueled by high doses of estrogen and progesterone. A closer look at pregnancy will help you understand the importance of sex hormones, how they work together, and how problems can arise.

Pregnancy involves millions and millions of cells dividing at high speed inside the body to create an entirely new human being. To survive and successfully complete a full-term pregnancy, a woman must have an immune system that will not destroy her baby while at the same time protecting her and her baby from invading germs. She requires a clotting system that allows blood to flow freely to her baby, while preventing her from hemorrhaging to death during birth. A pregnant woman needs breasts that will grow to the size of grapefruits in order to produce milk, and skin and ligaments that will stretch to accommodate the equivalent of two footballs. All of this is accomplished largely as the result of estrogen and progesterone working in sync.

Women's sex hormones have been carefully designed to work in a highly organized system with checks and balances. Estrogen is the creator; progesterone is the protector. It is almost Shakespearean. Estrogen stimulates eggs and cells to grow, promotes blood clotting, and helps to metabolize large amounts of cholesterol needed to make high levels of sex hormones. Estrogen raises serotonin levels to help attract mates and take care of babies lovingly. It moisturizes us and excites our sex drive so that we will make even more babies. It has even been suggested that estrogen makes women dress more colorfully to attract attention. It is as "out there" and powerful as a hormone can possibly be.

Progesterone, on the other hand, does nearly the reverse. It is the yin to estrogen's yang. Also known as the pregnancy hormone, progesterone is calming and sedating. It helps a pregnant woman to nest and rest. It induces sleep and quiets her mind. It prevents blood from overclotting and keeps a woman's body from taking on too much water and salt. It prevents breasts from growing too large and keeps the cells lining the uterus from growing too thick. Together, estrogen and progesterone sponsor pregnancy and maintain our balance as women.

Unfortunately, horse estrogen and synthetic imposters have replaced these multitalented hormones for more than seventy years. What is worse, in doing so they have tarnished the sterling reputation that our natural sex hormones deserve. Estrogen and progesterone, which have been circulating in the bodies of all females, have been deemed unfit and harmful. They have been accused of causing blood clots, heart disease, dementia, and cancer. Talk about ungrateful injustice.

The topic of female sex hormones has become almost political, and can divide a room. On one side are the staunch, in-your-face, ageless sex-goddess hormone supporters. You know them: the baby-booming, overachieving, double-tasking women who fell into menopause somewhere between infertility drugs and breast-feeding. They not only believe in hormones, they believe in lots of hormones—enough to keep you menstruating into your sixties and beyond. On the other side are the straight-laced hormone abolitionists who think estrogen is the work of the devil. Surely there is a middle ground, a place from which to look clearly through the mist of studies proclaiming doom and gloom for all hormones, synthetic and natural.

Unbalanced Sex Hormones: The Devil You Know

What is it like not to have enough sex hormones? Well, any hormonally deprived woman will tell you ("If she damn well feels like it!") that not having enough hormones is problematic. Put bluntly, it sucks.

Low Progesterone

Low progesterone usually means having a bloated belly and breasts that feel like overripe melons, heavy and tender to touch. Uncontrollable bitchiness may alternate with a moody sensation of low self-worth in a never-ending miserable loop in your mind. There can be erratic and often heavy bleeding that can leach your minerals, leave you exhausted, and make you cry. Without enough progesterone, sleep may become like a second job, with rituals, sleep aids, and prayers to the gods and goddesses for the blessing of some uninterrupted slumber.

Low Estrogen

Low estrogen usually involves hot flashes, dry eyes, dry mouth, dry vagina, dry skin, and even dry, slow bowels. Headaches are common. There is usually an abundance of wrinkled skin, and sagging breasts. Urinating can be a problem, with urinary leaks occurring involuntarily when sneezing, running, or laughing. You want to urinate too often, particularly at night. Orgasms seem like a thing of the past, and quite frankly, you may not even give a damn. Hair might be growing on your chin and falling out of your head. Your patience and calm demeanor are out the window; you want to harm people who are too slow or too simple-minded or too whatever.

What's Worse?

All these problems are the devil you know, and they are caused by too few sex hormones. But what if you know this and you are warned that if you want to do something to end your miseries, you risk having a stroke while recuperating from breast cancer in a dementia ward?

That's sort of how it feels these days. Which is worse, the devil you know or the devil you don't know?

First, let's be very specific about what we are calling hormones. Bioidentical hormones are identical in structure to what your body naturally produces. They behave the same and metabolize normally inside you. Synthetic hormones are not the same, and they behave and metabolize differently. For instance, Equilin (horse estrogen) breaks down into at least forty different foreign metabolites, some of which are hundreds of times stronger than our naturally occurring metabolites. That is what made Premarin so darn good: it is a very potent estrogen, much stronger than our naturally made estrogen. It is, after all, made by and strong enough for a horse. Many women feel very good when they take it, and it is still in use for this reason. Unfortunately, Equilin tends to form many cancer-promoting estrones (discussed in chapter 3), particularly 4-OH estrone, and when taken orally it increases blood clotting.

As you saw from my brief description of pregnancy, estrogen and progesterone are meant to work together. They oppose each other in a balanced way, and if you take one without the other, or if you use an imposter such as a synthetic hormone, you are bound to run into trouble. My mission is to help you to better understand your hormones, synthetic and natural, so that you can make sense of all the fearful reports and make an intelligent decision about using them to feel, look, and age better. The best decisions are made from a place of understanding, not fear.

When You Should Start: Perimenopause 101

Okay, so now that you know about how lousy low hormones can feel, let's look at when and how your hormones begin to drop. Perimenopause is tricky; it can sneak up on you when you least expect it. At first you have no idea that you are perimenopausal. Generally, somewhere in your thirties or forties, you may find that you're not sleeping well, particularly around your period. You may start to have PMS symptoms when you never did before. Most of the time, the symptoms of perimenopause are chalked up to being too tired, too busy, or just burned out.

Some call perimenopause the adolescence of old age. Remember how your body changed in puberty? Well, now it's happening in reverse, and it can be just as difficult and confusing. Like puberty, hormone levels are changing rapidly. One day they are up and the next day they are down. One day you feel sexual and energetic, and another day you are sexless and can't get out of bed. Puberty is over in three years, but for most women the hormonal ups and downs leading to menopause can last anywhere from five to fifteen years. Many women find that perimenopause is much more challenging than menopause itself. In menopause, hormone levels are low, but at least they are stable. During perimenopause, there is wide variability—day-to-day and month-to-month variability, which can feel as if your body is out of control. Sleep is erratic some days, sound others. Moods are up and down, and there is often a low-grade irritability and an unsettling dissatisfaction with everything around you. Your breasts may swell and your nipples can feel itchy or overly sensitive. Menstruation may be heavy and short one month, spotty or nonexistent the next.

Unfortunately, this is all taking place in our forties, when our careers are peaking, our lives changing. Often our children are in the throes of adolescence and our aging parents are in need of more care and time from us. During perimenopause it is not uncommon for marriages to be strained, or over, or beginning again for the second (or third) time. Perimenopause is busy, and we need to understand it to make it as easy on ourselves as possible. Whether you decide to use natural hormones or not, perimenopause is the time to understand progesterone.

Progesterone: The First Hormone to Fall

Progesterone is the first hormone to fall as women age, and the first sex hormone that I give to women. Progesterone is the perimenopausal hormone, and women need to realize its power and how to use it. Progesterone naturally prevents our breast and uterine cells from growing excessively. It regulates the menstrual cycle, reduces PMS symptoms, deepens sleep, lessens anxiety, reduces blood loss during menstruation, protects against blood clots, helps to maintain bone strength, enhances sleep, and prevents uterine fibroids and ovarian and breast cysts from forming. It also prevents hyperplasia and cancer from forming.

Without enough progesterone, estrogen runs wild, producing angry tempers, insomnia, anxiety, bloating, and heavy, unpredictable bleeding. A woman deprived of progesterone will have tender, swollen breasts and a thickened uterine lining.

"Raging hormones" pretty much sums up a woman lacking progesterone. Excessive bleeding is typical and can lead to anemia, D&C's, and surgeries for fibroids and cysts. Most hysterectomies are done for such problems, and many could be prevented by simply recognizing the symptoms of hormone imbalance (that is, lack of progesterone to balance estrogen) during perimenopause.

Our bodies were not designed erroneously. Our natural progesterone balances our estrogen's effects on our cells—preventing excess clotting and cell growth, in addition to the many effects noted above.

Progesterone Confusion

Progesterone is perhaps the most misunderstood hormone of all. Even worse, people are confusing it with its synthetic versions, which have many detrimental effects. The term "progestins" (also referred to as "progestogens" or "progestagens") refers to synthetic forms of progesterone. They are vastly different from natural progesterone in structure, function, and effects in your body. Progestins, not natural progesterone, have been clearly linked to breast cancer, heart disease, brain degeneration, depression, and blood clotting. Medroxyprogesterone (Provera) is the most common form of synthetic progesterone used in the United States and the form used in most of the mega-studies discussed in chapter 3.

Natural progesterone has been widely used in Europe. In addition to their appreciation for fine wine and cheeses, the French have recognized the merits of natural progesterone since 1980 and have published many studies demonstrating its safety and effectiveness. The one large U.S. study that used natural progesterone, known as the PEPI study and published in 1995, surprised researchers by showing that it improved lipids, unlike its synthetic counterpart. Unfortunately, natural progesterone drew criticisms of possibly predisposing to breast cancer (women using it had mammograms that were more dense). What these researchers failed to appreciate is that the dose used was too low (100 mg/day) to oppose the very strong synthetic horse estrogen used with it.

You may also come across other reports that claim there is no bene-fit to using transdermal bioidentical progesterone, but the doses used in these studies were also much too low (20 to 45 mg/day). Most women need 100 to 125 mg twice daily, orally or transdermally, to achieve ben-efits and protection.

Natural Progesterone Facts

Though progesterone was discovered more than seventy years ago, it has only recently been making headlines in scientific journals. An elo-quent 2007 article in *Endocrine Review* summarizes its many beneficial effects, such as its ability to reduce brain damage, limit stroke, and pre-vent Parkinson's disease, seizures, depression, memory loss, and even alcohol addiction. Here are some highlights from this and other scien-tific journals:

- Natural progesterone is made in a woman's brain throughout her lifetime. In menopause, even though blood levels of proges-terone fall to very low levels, brain levels fall by only 50 percent.
- Natural progesterone is metabolized into a metabolite (allopreg-nanolone) that improves insomnia, anxiety, depression, and mood changes associated with PMS symptoms, and protects the brain from degenerative diseases. Synthetic progesterones do not make this metabolite and consequently do not provide these same benefits.
- Natural progesterone acts as a diuretic, reducing bloating and weight gain. Synthetic progesterone acts conversely and is associ-ated with fluid retention, acne, weight gain, and migraine.
- Synthetic progesterones and their metabolites predispose to inflammation in blood vessels, and counteract beneficial effects of estradiol in the brain and heart. Natural progesterone does not.
- Synthetic progesterone increases heart-disease risk factors. It increases CRP and LDL (bad cholesterol), and reduces HDL (good cholesterol). Natural progesterone does not.
- All large hormone studies (including the WHI study, the Million Women Study, and the HERS study) clearly show an increase in breast cancer when using synthetic progesterone. No studies using natural progesterone and natural transdermal estradiol show this.

Early Perimenopause: PMS and Low Progesterone

Progesterone regulates your menstrual cycle. During perimenopause, the gradual decline in progesterone is the reason that your menstrual cycle begins to change. Usually the cycles get shorter. You may find that you are menstruating every 20 to 25 days, instead of every 28 to 30 days. Bleeding usually changes also; it gets heavier, or it may last longer and have larger clots. (Over time, as estrogen levels fall as well, the blood flow will again change, often becoming very light and crampy.)

Because your ovaries age at their own rate and on their own time frame, and you ovulate from a different ovary each month (left alternating with right), your symptoms will vary from month to month, too. Every other month you may have symptoms, or not. If you are ovulating from your stronger ovary one month, your cycle may be quite normal; when you ovulate from your weaker ovary the next month, your cycle may be shorter and your bleeding may be heavy or you may feel more emotional. This can become confusing: one month you are miserable, the next month you think, "Okay, I'm better"—only to be off-track again the following month. Once you realize what is actually going on, you can take charge of your body and symptoms and start to feel balanced again.

When to Use Progesterone

If you don't have enough progesterone, you will most likely notice PMS symptoms. You'll have some combination of breast pain and swelling, moodiness, depression, hand and ankle swelling, pimples, or even constipation before your period. The important thing is to notice when your symptoms are at their worst. Symptoms that are worse in the week or two before your period are due to low progesterone.

Most women feel great when their natural bioidentical progesterone is balanced, unlike when they use synthetics, which bring unpleasant side effects. Synthetic progesterone causes weight gain, swelling, sore breasts, and moody depressions; bioidentical progesterone does not. On bioidentical progesterone, my perimenopausal patients begin to sleep well; they become less moody and less bloated. Their cycles and bleeding return to normal. Occasionally, though, I will find a patient for whom progesterone just doesn't work. Such patients fare better on much lower doses or on herbal supports (vitex or Chinese herbs) or homeopathic progesterone—but more on that later.

How to Use Progesterone

The hardest part about using progesterone is timing. You may recall from your early sex education classes that every month (if pregnancy does not happen), your progesterone level will suddenly fall, giving rise to your menstrual bleeding. So when you are using progesterone, if you start it and forget to take it or simply stop taking it, you will bleed just as if you are having a period. You can start and stop estrogen without any problems, but if you start and stop progesterone you will, in most cases, spot or bleed. For this reason, progesterone use must be carefully timed with your menstrual cycle. If you are perimenopausal, it must be used in a cycled fashion or else erratic bleeding may occur. Erratic bleeding is not harmful but can certainly be annoying, confusing, and alarming.

Timing   Okay, here are the nuts and bolts of how to use progesterone to treat PMS and other symptoms of perimenopause. It's all about timing and dosages. The first day of your menstrual bleeding is considered "day 1." You need to know this day to know when to start using your progesterone. Use progesterone two weeks after your period starts (or two weeks after your period was due if you miss a cycle). Start progesterone on day 15 and stop it after day 25 of your cycle. Use it continuously for at least ten days. If you use progesterone during the first fifteen days, you will muck up your cycle; you will bleed erratically or not have a period at all. Once you stop your progesterone on day 25, you should expect to menstruate within two to four days. If you don't bleed within thirty days, lower the progesterone dose, next cycle. If your cycle is starting before day 27, you may need to increase the dose or start using progesterone a few days earlier, say on day 13 or 14.

Dosages   Progesterone is not generally an easy hormone to absorb. I recommend using it twice daily. Most women absorb progesterone from the skin well, but some have difficulty even with a high-dose cream. You'll know that you are absorbing well if your symptoms improve. If your cycles are still heavy, too short, or erratic, check a progesterone blood level while on the cream (or check a twenty-four-hour urine pregnanediol level). Remember not to use a saliva level if you are using cream or lotion; the level will be (falsely) high. If your blood level is too low (under 6 ng/ml), either increase the dose or add an oral dose at bedtime.

Most women need somewhere between 100 and 125 mg of transdermal progesterone twice daily, or 200 to 300 mg orally at bedtime. If you use transdermal progesterone, apply it to the inner and outer arm (one arm, both sides, rubbed in well) or to the abdomen. If you are experiencing breast tenderness, have breast cysts, or have breast calcifications on your mammograms, then apply some leftover progesterone cream from your hand directly onto your breasts. Often the blood supply inside breast cysts or nodules is poor, and a small amount of hormone cream helps. If you are overweight, it is best to avoid abdominal or thigh applications, as absorption will be poor. In that case, I recommend oral progesterone first.

Remember, if your symptoms are not improving or you are not sure you are absorbing the progesterone after checking a level and increasing your dose, switch to oral progesterone.

Fine-Tuning   Normally the regimen I just described works really well, and your cycle will be restored and regulated. You will also be protecting your bones from bone loss, and you will be protecting your breasts and uterus from any raging estrogen your body is still making. You have to stay flexible with your progesterone program. There are times when you will want to fine-tune. For example:

A Short Cycle   If you are using progesterone and your menstrual cycle is too short—that is, you are bleeding every twenty to twenty-five days—the first thing to consider is whether you are taking enough progesterone. You should discuss this with your doctor and increase your dose or measure your blood level of progesterone when you are on it. No one really knows the ideal blood level for progesterone, but most ovulating women have a level between 5 and 12 ng/ml after they ovulate. (You need a level of around 11 ng/ml to get pregnant.) So I aim for a level between 6 and 12 ng/ml in my patients. If your level is okay, then take a half dose of progesterone earlier in the cycle, say around days 10 through 14, and increase to full strength on days 13 to 25, to help lengthen your cycle.

A Long Cycle   If your cycle is too long (greater than thirty days) or your period is not coming until five days or more after stopping the progesterone, you may need to lower your dose. Using too much could delay your period.

You Don't Want to Stop   If you feel "sooooooo good" on the progesterone—if your mood and sleep are much better on progesterone and you feel as though you want to be on some every day—you can start using a low dose (50 mg) on days 7 to 10 and gradually increase the dose to 100 mg for days 10 to 13. Then use a full dose (200 to 300 mg) on days 14 to 25.

Progesterone Preparations

Progesterone can be taken safely orally or as a skin cream; it can even be taken as both—skin cream in the morning and an oral capsule at bedtime.

Bioidentical natural progesterone is available (1) in pill form; (2) by cream, gel, or lotion applied to the skin; (3) as a cream or suppository in the vagina; and (4) by injection. Deciding which form of progesterone to use depends on cost, symptoms, and sometimes a little trial and error.

Pills and Creams   With oral progesterone sleepiness is a common side effect, so I prescribe it at bedtime if there are sleep problems. If you take it orally during the day, it will cause drowsiness or laziness. Most women report much deeper sleep while on oral progesterone. About 10 percent of my patients become irritable or feel hung over when using oral progesterone. If this happens to you, switch to a compounded skin cream or lotion.

I prefer using topical progesterone skin cream or lotion because it also promotes a good night's sleep and tends to have fewer side effects. Side effects are not common with natural progesterone compared with synthetic progesterone, but some women become depressed or irritable on it. These potential side effects are more common with oral forms. Very rarely, women show "paradoxical" symptoms—that is, they become more excited or their insomnia worsens on progesterone because their body converts it into cortisol, a stimulating hormone. (I have only seen this happen once.) About 10 percent of my patients get irritable with oral progesterone. I'm one of them, so I switched to transdermal progesterone and have experienced no side effects; in fact, it makes me feel great.

Many insurance companies will cover progesterone pills and com-pounded progesterone transdermal skin lotion. Prescription proges-terone is marketed as Prometrium and comes in 100 mg and 200 mg oral doses (the typical dose is 100 to 300 mg nightly). Because Prometrium is made with a peanut oil suspension, it cannot be used if you have a peanut allergy. Compounding pharmacies can make any form of bioidentical progesterone without peanut oil and in individualized doses. Proges-terone creams and oral tablets can be used together: tablets at night to help deepen sleep, and cream in the morning to ensure that progesterone lasts all day without the drowsy side effects of pills.

There are wild yam (*Dioscorea*) and soy-based progesterone creams available over the counter in many health food stores, which do not require a prescription. Wild yam has a mild progesterone effect, but it does not raise your body's own progesterone level. This may be fine for young women with mild PMS symptoms, but for most of us older per-imenopausal women it won't be strong enough. Most over-the-counter creams have only very small amounts of progesterone (10 to 20 mg per tsp), and many may not have any progesterone at all. Such creams are not standardized, and the progesterone content varies quite a bit. Many over-the-counter creams also contain methylparaben and related sub-stances that have been linked to breast cancer. You certainly wouldn't want to put these creams directly onto your breasts, so it's important to know all of the chemicals used in any transdermal preparation, whether over-the-counter or compounded. Read labels and ask your pharmacist to be sure creams/lotions are paraben-free.

Vaginal Preparations   Vaginal preparations are usually used in cases where the uterus is in need of high doses of progesterone, such as infer-tility or uterine hyperplasia (overactive lining of the uterus, often with bleeding). From time to time with a patient who simply gets too depressed on progesterone, I prescribe progesterone vaginally. This provides the uterine benefits of progesterone without any possible moody side effects. A 2007 animal study showed that vaginal progesterone provided protection from estrogen effects to the breasts and uterine lining just as well as oral progesterone. Vaginal progesterone can be compounded into vaginal suppositories or cream, and I typically prescribe 100 to 200 mg daily during the ten days before the period (days 15 to 25).

Vaginal progesterone is available by prescription as FDA-approved Crinone gel (4 percent or 8 percent) and is applied with a vaginal insert. This can be a bit messy, and most of my patients prefer to use compounded vaginal suppositories. Progesterone is not harmful to men in the way that estrogen can be, so if you are on it while having sexual relations, there is no worry of transferring progesterone to your partner. (Sometimes I prescribe very low doses of progesterone to men with insomnia, hair loss, or anxiety.)

Injectable Progesterone

Injectable progesterone is usually only used to treat infertility or to prevent miscarriage. It was the only form of progesterone available before 1980, when pharmacists discovered how to suspend progesterone in oil.

Hormones? Supplements? Everything?

There are many effective herbal and vitamin supports that can dramatically improve hormone balance and, in particular, progesterone levels. Such treatments have been used effectively for centuries in both the East and the West. Supporting clinical studies abound.

Supplements can play an important role in improving hormone metabolism in your liver and bowels. The symptoms of PMS, which according to Chinese medicine, are due to a stagnant liver (discussed in chapter 3), respond well to herbal supplements, glandular extracts, and vitamins and mineral supplements. It is always preferable to obtain vitamins and minerals from your food; but often, despite the best intentions, great foods may not be enough. As you age, your digestion and ability to absorb nutrients deteriorate. Alcohol, caffeine, and certain medications, such as birth control pills, deplete your vitamins and minerals and stress your liver metabolism. Excess stress and excessive bleeding can worsen things further.

I do not advocate using the same vitamins or minerals continuously because, over time, constant dosing of one particular vitamin or mineral can cause toxicity. Below are some suggestions for herbs, vitamins, and minerals to alleviate many complaints of perimenopause. You can try these before starting on hormones or in conjunction with hormone support.

To avoid PMS symptoms, such as breast pain and swelling, moodiness, headache, nausea, and constipation during the first two weeks before your period, you must have adequate progesterone and good metabolism in your liver. Here are some remedies to improve progesterone levels and liver metabolism of hormones:

1. **Chasteberry** (*vitex agnus-castus*), or monk's pepper, has been used for hundreds of years for women's health issues such as infertility, breast pain, heavy bleeding, and PMS symptoms. It does this by increasing levels of progesterone (via the brain's pituitary hormone, LH, or luteinizing hormone). It also increases dopamine levels and lowers prolactin. I find this herb most useful during the early years of perimenopause, when progesterone levels are beginning to decline. As your egg supplies dwindle in the later years of perimenopause, vitex becomes less effective, since your ovaries eventually lose their ability to respond to any brain hormone stimulation. Some doctors caution against using vitex with progesterone, but I have not seen any problems in my patients using both. However, the need for both is a sign that your ovaries are no longer responding to the vitex as well, and you should consider switching to progesterone alone. Dosages vary depending on the concentration of your herbal tincture. (You may be wondering why they call it *chaste*berry if it helps make women fertile. When given to a man, it reduces his sexual desire by increasing his progesterone level—which is why it is also called monk's pepper.)

2. **Liver nutrients** can be used, but not every day and not forever. I typically prescribe the following for the two weeks before the period:

      Milk Thistle or Lipotropic complex (a combination of liver herbs such as dandelion root [*taraxacum officinale*], Chelidonium, beet leaf, black radish with methionine and inositol, vitamin B_6 and B_{12}). Doses depend on the strength of the extracts. Typically 400 to 500 mg of milk thistle two to three times daily are used.

Beta-sitosterol (500 to 800 mg/day) helps improve estrogen metabolism and can provide relief from breast pain.

Chinese herbal blends exist in numerous recipes and are available in any Chinatown or from a Chinese herbalist. One such blend, Free and Easy Powder, is commonly used by women in China for most premenstrual complaints.

Acupuncture is not a liver nutrient, but it is an effective treatment for improving liver function. It works well for most symptoms of PMS. I usually recommend treating in the week or two before the period for best results.

3. **B vitamins** can alleviate symptoms of PMS and are also used for treating moodiness and depression. B vitamins are difficult to measure effectively, as they exist primarily inside cells, but there are tests (organic acid tests and metabolic profiles) that can determine if B vitamin metabolism is working well inside your cells. The most important B vitamins for women's health are vitamins B_6, B_{12}, and folic acid. These three nutrients are needed to process estrogen and to make melatonin and other neurotransmitters, such as SAMe (S-adenosyl methionine) or GABA (gamma-aminobutyric acid). Oral estrogen and birth control pills lower these vitamin levels. I recommend using a B complex (100 mg/day). If you prefer to take them separately, the usual dose for B_6 is 50 mg twice daily. There is an activated form of vitamin B_6 called P5P (pyridoxal-5-phosphate), which can be easier for your body to utilize. For folic acid, the usual dose is 0.8 to 2 mg a day. Some women have difficulty methylating B_{12} and folic acid and need a methylated vitamin. Usual doses for B_{12} are 1,000 mcg daily (but much higher doses will be needed if you have a genetic polymorphism that limits methylation). Both B_{12} and folic acid are safe and literally impossible to overdose.

4. **Essential fatty acids (omega-3 and omega-6 oils)** Many women are deficient in essential fatty acids. Several studies have shown high-dose omega-3 oils to be as effective as antidepressants for

treating depression. Omega-6 fatty acids may also have a role in treating PMS. The omega-6 metabolite GLA (gamma-linolenic acid) has been shown to be deficient in women with PMS. Interestingly, GLA production requires vitamins B_6, magnesium, and zinc, all known to help PMS symptoms. Evening primrose oil, borage oil, and black currant oil contain large amounts of GLA and are used in PMS. To date studies using GLA oils did not significantly improve mood, but they have been shown to relieve breast pain. I recommend varying your omega-3 oils (flax oil, fish oil, cod liver oil, or krill oil) every two to three months with the GLA-rich omega-6 oils mentioned above (2,000 to 5,000 mg/day).

5. **Adrenal supports** will be discussed more fully in chapter 10, but it is important to understand that your adrenal glands are designed to produce your sex hormones as you age. If you are experiencing a lot of perimenopausal symptoms, you will want to strengthen your adrenals so that they can better serve you. DHEA and pregnenolone are important adrenal hormones, and levels of these hormones should be maintained in the mid to upper-middle ranges. Adrenal extracts and herbs such as Panax Ginseng, Siberian Ginseng, Rhodiola, and Ashwaganda help to do this. They are discussed in chapter 10.

6. **Dong quai** (*angelica sinesis*) is an ancient Asian herb and a mainstay of most Chinese women's formulas. Much like soy, Dong quai has an estrogen-regulating effect. It will enhance estrogenic effects when estrogen levels are low, and reduce its effects when estrogen levels are too high. According to Chinese medicine, it is used to nourish the blood and treat scanty periods, anemia, and menstrual cramps. In addition, it appears to ward off yeast infections and can help reduce PMS symptoms. It is always used in conjunction with other herbs in Chinese formulas. For this reason, clinical trials with this herb alone have not proved its effectiveness. Nonetheless, it has been used successfully for more than two thousand years for many women's health problems.

7. **Vitamin E** has been shown to reduce fibrocystic breast symptoms. In general, antioxidants such as vitamin E support hormone production, and studies have shown vitamin E to be effective in reducing breast pain and hot flashes. Typically, moderate doses (800 U/day) are needed. There are two primary forms

of vitamin E: alpha tocopherol and gamma tocopherol. For hormonal health, I generally recommend using a mixed tocopherol, a combination of both.

8. **Magnesium** is needed for nearly every energy-producing function in your body, and it is vital for helping your system cope with stress. Magnesium deficiency is rampant. It is the most common mineral deficiency that I see in my patients. Low magnesium will cause fatigue, headache, irritability, and depression. An RBC magnesium test will tell you your level, but don't request a routine serum level, as this will not show a deficiency unless your level is very low (by this time you would be at risk of developing a heart arrhythmia). The ideal RBC magnesium level should be greater than 4.8 mg/dL (with normal ranges reported at 4.0 to 6.4 mg/dL).

I often prescribe magnesium with taurine, an amino acid that helps to ensure that magnesium will enter your cells, where it is needed. Taurine is also frequently low, and it can be measured with a fasting blood test. If you have had prolonged depression or chronic yeast infections, you are probably low in taurine. Often it's impossible to correct low magnesium without taurine (1,000 to 2,000 mg/day). Both magnesium and taurine are calming and can help you to sleep, so I often recommend taking them at bedtime, or during the day if there is anxiety.

If the supplements discussed above help you, great; but if you are still struggling, you should consider cycling natural progesterone and adding estrogen (see chapter 9) when and if you need it.

Summary: Taking Care of Yourself in Perimenopause

The symptoms of perimenopause (PMS, insomnia, and anxiety before your period; heavy bleeding; short, irregular cycles) are mainly about lack of progesterone. Over time, you may develop low estrogen symptoms, too (headaches, fatigue, depression, loss of sex drive, hot flashes—initially worse when menstruating or when just finished menstruating), which are discussed in chapter 9.

Here are three things you can do to help perimenopausal symptoms in general:

1. **Look at your lifestyle and stress levels.** Any activities that help to nurture you and reduce stress can help to support hormone production. Activities such as yoga, exercise, meditation, adequate rest/relaxation, acupuncture, body work, and taking care of chronic conditions (including dental infections, chronic pain, chronic yeast, toxic exposures) will help.
2. **Talk to a doctor about your symptoms.** Decide if you should measure your hormones to determine if hormone deficiency is the cause of your symptoms. Measure progesterone when it peaks, on days 19 to 21 of your cycle. Measure estrogen when it is lowest, during your period, in the week following your period, or when your symptoms are most severe.
3. **Look at your diet.** Aim for eight combined servings of fresh (preferably organic) fruits and vegetables every day. Avoid dairy, excess sugar, caffeine, alcohol, and processed foods. Use herbs and vitamin supplements judiciously (in a rotated fashion, varying supplements every three to four months) to support your hormones and to help stabilize changing levels (see below).

If symptoms are mainly in the week or two before your period and you have tried everything above without success, or you're just too busy, lazy, or overwhelmed to do these things, ask your doctor to start you on natural progesterone.

If your symptoms are happening all over the place, in no clear relationship to your cycle, or if you are skipping periods, test and treat for low estradiol. See chapter 9 for more discussion of sex hormones.

Sandy: Liver Herbs and Hormones in Perimenopause

Sandy was forty-six years old when I first met her. She had developed problems that no one could figure out. She had intermittent nausea and pain in her upper right belly. She'd had all of the usual tests—upper G.I. series, liver function tests, and a gallbladder ultrasound. She was told repeatedly that she was fine, but she still had symptoms.

On questioning, she told me that her symptoms were always

worse when she drank coffee and before her period. Her periods were regular, but she had breast swelling and tenderness for nearly two weeks before her period. Headaches and moodiness were coming on in the days before her cycle, but she understood that this was "normal." Her blood flow had become heavy and more crampy, and her bleeding was somewhat erratic—spotting, then heavy with cramps, followed by a day of no bleeding and then more spotting. When I examined her, her Chinese pulses were very weak and choppy, her hair was thinning, her face and fingers looked puffy, and she had tenderness around her upper belly on both sides.

Blood tests showed a mild anemia and a low-normal magnesium of 4.4 ng/dL (the normal range is 4.0 to 6.4 ng/dL). I explained to her that an RBC magnesium less than 4.8 could be contributing to her menstrual cramps, fatigue, headaches, and poor hormone function. She didn't really think of herself as perimenopausal, and she didn't like the idea that she might need hormones, something she expected to deal with only when she was older (or perhaps not at all). So we decided to treat her with herbs and vitamins.

No Western medical test showed liver or gallbladder disease, but from a Chinese medical standpoint, her symptoms indicated a classic case of liver stagnation (with deficiency). She had very typical signs of low progesterone, with her symptoms all worse before her period—heavy, tender breasts, fluid retention, and heavy menstrual flow. Her symptoms were a combination of low progesterone and liver *qi* stagnation with deficiency.

I started her on a lipotropic complex and the Chinese formula for PMS (Xiao Yao San). I also gave her NAC, B complex, calcium, magnesium, and iron supplements. A couple of months later, she reported that her pain and nausea had improved almost immediately, and she only had breast swelling every other month. She was still moody before her period, but it was less intense. Her cycles were still coming early, by day 26, and though the flow seemed better (fewer clots and no starting and stopping), it was still heavy.

We decided to add progesterone cream to help lessen her blood loss; she couldn't afford to keep losing minerals every month. She started on a cream (100 mg twice daily) that she applied to her belly on days 15 through 25.

After one cycle she called to say that her sleep was great but her cycle was still short and heavy, and she was still irritable. So we increased her cream to 125 mg twice daily, and within two months her cycle had normalized.

Sheila Part 1: Herbs and Progesterone

Sheila was a forty-five-year-old woman with PMS. She normally enjoyed life until the middle of her cycle hit, and then her personality took a dive. Each month she would become angry, irritable, impatient, weepy, and tearful. She couldn't seem to help herself. She'd been doing yoga and meditating, which helped, but after a few hours she was back to misery.

Her periods were "fine" and regular, but she did notice bloating in her belly with constipation that was worse before her period. Otherwise she had no real complaints. Her sleep and energy were okay. Her exam was normal, but her blood tests showed a very low RBC magnesium 3.6 (4.2 to 6.8 mg/dL), no anemia but a low-normal ferritin 28 (10 to 300 ng/ml), and a normal thyroid. So Sheila began replacing her magnesium and using a good multivitamin with iron. I recommended that she use vitamin B_6 with some Chinese liver herbs and referred her to an acupuncturist in the week or two before her period.

She did well on this regimen, but after a few months she came to see me complaining of heavy periods and loose stools. I reminded her that magnesium could cause her stools to be too loose, so we changed her magnesium supplement from magnesium citrate, which had alleviated her constipation, to magnesium glycinate, which doesn't usually affect the bowels. I told her she could go back on magnesium citrate in the future if she ever became constipated again. Her heavy periods, I explained, were most likely due to progesterone deficiency, and she agreed to try the herb vitex to see if her progesterone levels would improve.

A couple of cycles later she reported that her PMS was completely gone and her cycles were less heavy. Over the ensuing years, as Sheila traversed perimenopause, she would still develop symptoms, particularly when her rocky relationship tanked or her mother became ill, but she knew what to do. If PMS flared, she knew to restart her Chinese herbs, which she referred to as "bitch pills," and she would take vitamin B$_6$ and some omega-3 and omega-6 oils (flax oil and/or evening primrose oil), which also helped her constipation. She had refused to give up her coffee and still ate erratically, but she knew to manage her "angry liver" with lipotropic complex and acupuncture. If her sleep became a problem, she would take some tryptophan (5HTP, 50 to 100 mg) at bedtime or a small dose of melatonin (0.5 mg). She was a woman aware and in control of her symptoms. After her forty-sixth birthday, her cycles started to shorten and get heavy again on the vitex, which she had taken erratically, so I switched her to progesterone cream. On this, her cycles become regular—that is, for a while. . . . (to be continued in chapter 9).

Sex Hormones Part 2: Using Bioidentical Estrogen and Testosterone

Perimenopause gradually morphs into menopause. All women experience this transition differently, but the physiology is the same for all of us. Gradually, our ovaries age, producing less and less estrogen, progesterone, and testosterone. Chapter 8 focused on progesterone, which falls first in the early stages of perimenopause. In the later stages, estrogen falls, with testosterone sputtering along in a much smaller capacity. This chapter will tell you how to support estrogen and testosterone naturally and safely. But first, here is some introductory biology to set the stage and help you understand why you feel the way you do.

How Your Ovaries Age

Ovarian decline is not a sudden process. Your ovaries have been on the decline, physiologically, since you were born. On the first day of your life you had somewhere between 1 to 2 million eggs in your ovaries. Every day since then your egg supply has been gradually dwindling. By the time you hormonally peaked as a teenager, your egg count was down to a mere 400,000, (talk about ticking clocks). After that, with every menstrual cycle, under the control of your brain's pituitary hormone FSH (follicle stimulating hormone), one of your ovaries miraculously created an egg (from a thousand potential follicles). Under the influence of another brain hormone, LH (luteinizing hormone), this lucky egg was released into your inner world for (possibly) the adventure of a lifetime, quite literally. An ongoing mini-Olympics occurred monthly inside your body for roughly thirty-five years and then gradually came to an end, but not without some physiologic pomp and ceremony.

As your ovaries age, they become more independent and unwilling to respond at the whim of your brain hormones. FSH and LH seem to lose their power. These two hormones climb to higher and higher levels in an effort to get some ovarian response, some eggs to release. Eventually, your ovaries just plain quit. After years of faithful service, they've had enough. But that's not the case with your brain hormones. FSH and LH persist at high levels throughout menopause, while your ovaries go on a well-deserved retirement, no longer producing monthly cycles of progesterone or estrogen, and leisurely chugging out about one-half as much testosterone. We can learn from this aging process.

What Is Estrogen?

Before we go into too much detail about how to use estrogen, let's talk about what she is exactly. You know from chapter 3 that your natural estrogen is not the same as horse estrogen found in mare's urine, but there are many misconceptions about natural estrogen. Personally, I love the fact that she is so mysterious, changeable, poorly understood, and hard to pin down. She is, after all, the personification of all female archetypes and what gives us our female mystique. Reports on estrogen used to be good; lately they have been shrouded in gloom. The press has given estrogen a doomsday hype, and all that is good about her has been lost. As always, there are two sides to every story. When it comes to estrogen, most of us are familiar with only one. Trust me, she is not the Wicked Witch of the West, as the headlines would lead you to believe.

To help make things clear, here are some general facts about estrogen:

- Our own natural estrogen is *not* simply one hormone; it is a family of hormones—some weak, some strong, some sexy, some protective, and some dangerous.
- Whenever you speak of natural estrogen, know that you are speaking of at least three circulating estrogens and at least five active estrogen metabolites (and many more if you're talking about synthetic estrogen).
- All hormones work together in a carefully balanced system. Estrogen is stimulating to our mind and our cells and has a tendency to promote blood clotting. Progesterone naturally opposes estrogen. It is calming, limits cell growth, and lessens blood clotting.
- Even if you don't take estrogen, your body continues to make it. All women face a risk of developing breast cancer whether they use estrogen or not.
- The more overweight you are, the more estrogen you will make, increasing your risk of developing breast cancer, gallbladder disease, and blood clots.
- Your estrogens can interconvert into either active, dangerous metabolites or benign breakdown products—depending on your genes, diet, and environment.
- As you enter menopause, your ovaries stop producing the strongest estrogen, estradiol, but your body produces higher levels of a weaker, potentially carcinogenic estrogen, estrone. This change is responsible for most of the symptoms of menopause.
- Low estradiol levels result in an increase in heart disease, bone loss, dementia, depression, sexual dysfunction, and hair thinning.
- There are at least five types of estrones. High levels of certain estrones (4-OH estrone and 16-OH estrone) have been linked to cancer.
- Some forms of estrogen (estriol, 2-hydroxyestrone, and 2-methoxyestrone) appear to prevent breast cancer and bone loss and to lower your risk of heart disease.

All about the Estrogen Family

Estrogen is a family of hormones with three major circulating forms: E1 (estrone), E2 (estradiol), and E3 (estriol), each playing a different role. Research in the estrogen family is still relatively young.

Estrone (E1)

Estrone is the major form of estrogen made by your body during menopause. Estrone levels increase as estradiol production falls during perimenopause and menopause. Estrones are produced mainly in your liver and fat cells, but not in your ovaries, which wind down during perimenopause.

Most of your estrogen metabolizes into some form of estrone. Now, there's really no such thing as a good or bad hormone, but bad estrones are a bit like hazardous waste, as they can pollute the body by causing cell damage if the body doesn't handle them properly. Because estrones are produced in the fat cells, overweight women tend to have higher levels of estrone than thin women, which explains why overweight women have more estrogen-related problems, such as gallbladder disease, fibroids, uterine hyperplasia, and even breast cancer.

I don't prescribe estrone in menopause since there is already too much estrone compared with estradiol, but I do monitor the different types of estrones with twenty-four-hour urine tests to ensure that a woman is metabolizing her estrogen in a safe manner (see chapter 3). Check your estrone levels at least one time each year while you are using estrogen support. This is especially important if you have a family history of breast, uterine, ovarian, or even prostate cancer. These cancers are all connected to faulty estrogen metabolism, and you can inherit a tendency to produce bad estrones.

Estradiol (E2)

Estradiol is the "va-va-va-voom" form of estrogen. It is sexy and strong and what being a woman is all about. Estradiol is the major estrogen made by the ovaries before menopause. It gives women their joie de vivre feeling. It is the form I recommend that all women start with. Without enough estradiol, a woman's life seems dull, flat, dry, and sexless. Estradiol is the most important natural antidepressant in women, superior to any prescription antidepressant because, while lifting your mood (by increasing your serotonin levels), it enhances your sex drive and strengthens your bones, skin, and hair. It helps you to sleep longer and deeper, and moisturizes your skin, lips, eyes, and vagina—basically every mucous membrane in your body. Even constipation symptoms can improve with estradiol support.

Estriol (E3)

Estriol is the weakest of the circulating estrogens, and the major form of estrogen in your body during pregnancy, when it is made by your baby's placenta. When you're not pregnant, it is made mostly in your liver and breast cells (from 16 OH-estrone, discussed in chapter 3). It is a unique form of estrogen, because it does not appear to break down into any other metabolite. Yet, its exact purpose (aside from its role in pregnancy) is unclear. It seems to provide benefits similar to estradiol, but in a much weaker form, being about one-eighth as strong. It may have a role in regulating estrogen, because it attaches to the estrogen receptors on cells, but it does not do too much to the cells. Some believe it may act like an "estrogen policewoman," determining which cells are turned on or off to estrogen.

Studies have shown that women with breast cancer typically have lower than normal levels of estriol. It is also known that women who have been pregnant, and thereby exposed to high estriol levels, are less likely to develop breast cancer. For these reasons, and because estriol does not form harmful estrogen metabolites (as far as we know), it has been postulated that estriol is a safer form of estrogen that may help prevent breast cancer. These theories are logical but unproven. I use estriol, but only after I have prescribed estradiol and tested to see if my patient needs estriol. I also use estriol to treat vaginal dryness, and it may be the preferred estrogen to use in women who have a history of breast cancer, but more on all this later.

A Lifetime of Estrogen Ups and Downs

As a teenager your ovaries made vast amounts of estradiol, enough to make you giggle, shriek, and flirt, and think all day about whom you liked and who liked you. You daydreamed about sex and had enough energy to stay out late. You were at your fertile peak and the world was your oyster. Because estradiol is lowest during your period and the ensuing week, you may have had your first taste of low estradiol as the menstrual blues, or as menstrual headaches or cramps.

In the weeks or months after childbirth, you may have felt a more prolonged effect of low estradiol, manifesting as postpartum depression or simply no interest in sex or getting dressed up. As you ate well, rested, weaned, and started menstruating once again, your estradiol should have come back on track.

Low estradiol symptoms can hit you at other times, like after a tubal ligation (tying your tubes) or pelvic surgery (for fibroid or ovarian cysts), because the blood supply to the ovaries can be affected. You could have a simple procedure and not understand why the next few weeks feel like someone died. In addition, birth control pills, though filled with (synthetic) hormones, lower your available estradiol levels (as well as cortisol and testosterone) and can leave you feeling habitually down.

By the time you hit your late thirties to early forties you might notice all the symptoms we discussed in chapter 8 as a result of falling progesterone, with PMS, insomnia, and possibly bleeding problems. But it is not until the late stages of perimenopause that low estradiol gives you symptoms.

Because estrogen is lowest during your period and the week after, symptoms of low estradiol tend to occur here first, during perimenopause. So, in addition to PMS symptoms from your waning progesterone, you may over time start to develop menstrual headaches, depression, fatigue, or sharp menstrual cramps during and immediately after your period. You may notice that where you used to feel great once your period came, you are now tired and depressed throughout your cycle. Some women feel like they have entered a state of constant PMS. When I hear this from a patient, I know that her progesterone is down and that her estradiol has begun to fall, too.

Unfortunately, most women don't fully appreciate what's happening until hot flashes appear. When they do finally realize that their hormones are out of whack, they may have already developed a dependency on sleeping pills (which are probably no longer working) and they're usually experiencing weight gains from their antidepressants. Even worse, they may be suffering the physical effects of waning hormones: memory lapses, bone loss, uterine fibroids or breast cysts, and a rise in lipids, blood pressure, or other markers of heart disease. Many women come to me too late, when they are hemorrhaging and needing hysterectomies for large fibroids that developed as a result of years of unrecognized progesterone deficiency. Many have undergone biopsies for breast lumps. This is why it's important to recognize your symptoms early during perimenopause and treat underlying progesterone and estrogen deficiency promptly.

Symptoms of Low Estrogen

The low estrogen symptoms described above can arise at any age. Symptoms usually start when your estradiol level falls too low. I have a saying: "Never argue with a woman who has an estradiol level below 60 pg/ml, you won't win. And you will regret ever trying." Estradiol is one of the most important driving forces in a woman's body and psyche because it supports serotonin, the neurotransmitter needed to experience joy, peace, and even good sex. Without it a woman can become humorless, dark, and disinterested in love.

Low Estradiol, Low Serotonin

Low estradiol and low serotonin is the root of many perimenopausal and menopausal symptoms. Low serotonin may cause headaches, depression, fatigue, a lower sex drive, insomnia, and hot flashes. When serotonin levels fall, your body compensates by raising other neurotransmitters such as norepinephrine. Norepinephrine is normally balanced with the adrenal hormone epinephrine (adrenaline). If you are under stress, or if your adrenals are weak, you will not have good epinephrine levels. It is believed that an imbalance between norepinephrine and epinephrine (too much norepinephrine and not enough epineph-rine to balance it) is largely responsible for hot flashes, palpitations, insomnia, and anxiety commonly seen during perimenopause and menopause. That is how antidepressants (SSRIs) work to help menopausal symptoms: they "raise" serotonin. But these treatments, though effective and useful temporarily, are not treating the root cause, low estradiol. Such treatments do not actually increase your serotonin stores, they simply block the breakdown of serotonin in your body, so your body experiences higher serotonin levels. Over time, deficiency of serotonin and other neurotransmitters, such as dopamine, may occur, leading to more depression and a lower sex drive. In addition, antide-pressants will not protect you from what is happening to your bones, lipids, and blood vessels as a result of low estradiol.

Other Low Estrogen Symptoms

We are all familiar with the classic symptoms of low estrogen men-tioned above, but there are many less well known, equally miserable symptoms, such as migraines, sharp menstrual cramps, dry eyes, dry mouth, cough, constipation, joint pains (particularly the thumbs), fre-quent urination, urinary and vaginal infections, and poor bladder con-trol. All this can occur if your estradiol level falls below 60 pg/ml. Without enough estrogen, fine lines begin to appear on your face, par-ticularly around your mouth, eyes, and forehead. Breasts tend to shrink and sag and feel less responsive sexually. A woman's estradiol is the pri-mary hormone responsible for her libido, or sex drive. In general, low estradiol can make you feel dried up, tired, hot, irritable, unattractive, and depressed.

Low Estrogen in Perimenopause

Most women don't think they need estrogen if they are cycling and don't have hot flashes. But as you learn more about your symptoms, you will recognize when your estrogen starts to change. I recommend that women start estrogen support early, when mood, sleep, and energy levels are first affected. You want to start using it before you lose bone, develop heart risk factors, or suffer depression or sexual dysfunction.

Perimenopause is a safe time to use estradiol; you are normally producing estradiol naturally at this time anyway.

During perimenopause, your period will help to tell you about how your estrogen levels are doing. As your estrogen falls, usually your menstrual blood flow becomes less heavy and darker, and you bleed fewer days, usually only two or three. Often when this happens, women notice new symptoms such as headaches and sharp cramps. But some women, particularly those who are anemic or have fibroids or low thyroid problems, can bleed heavily despite low levels of estrogen.

Skipping Cycles

If you start to skip cycles, things can feel very confusing, particularly if you've always been regular. The reason that you skip cycles is because your right and left ovaries age at different rates, not because your body is going haywire. One ovary may produce fewer hormones than the other and skip, while the other is working normally. So you will think you are having a long, perhaps fifty-day cycle, when you are really having two cycles—a "normal" one from your less-aged ovary (a normal bleed), alternating the next month with your weaker ovary, which won't make enough estrogen to bleed, so the cycle appears to be fifty to sixty days long. It is important to recognize this so you won't feel so out of control. It will also help you decide when to cycle your progesterone (discussed below). Eventually, one day your cycles will stop altogether, whether you use support or not.

Transitioning into Menopause

Menopause is defined in the medical books as "the absence of a menstrual period for twelve months." It is a retrospective definition. That is, no doctor will tell you that you are there until you've lost your period for one full year. But trust me, once your last standing ovary is sputtering, your periods are happening every three to six months, and you are waking hot and sweaty, you are surely in menopause and woe betide anyone who tries telling you otherwise. In fact, it is my considered opinion that no one should tell any woman with such an array of symptoms anything she doesn't want to hear.

Most women are destined to spend one-half of their lifetime in menopause. Although it is a time of great changes, most women actually start to feel better and less volatile as compared with perimenopause. The hormonal ups and downs and erratic bleeding end and stability reigns. Menopause is the time to take stock of your health and take a hard look at supporting estrogen, at least for the first decade of menopause.

Health Changes in Menopause

Menopause is busy. The possible consequences of losing progesterone, estradiol, serotonin, and one-half of your testosterone, in addition to gaining extra estrones, can have an enormous impact physiologically. You are more prone to breast cancer, weight gain, high cholesterol, high blood pressure, heart disease, bone loss, memory loss, hair loss, dry skin, and wrinkles. It is a lot of potential losses. This is the time to be proactive.

So here is what I recommend to evaluate your health risks:

- Obtain a bone density test, if you haven't already done this. Most women lose more bone in the first few years of menopause than at any other time.
- Have a mammogram every year. (You should have been having mammograms every year after the age of forty, as recommended by the American Cancer Institute.)
- All women should have a Pap smear every year to monitor HPV (human papilloma virus), which is associated with cervical cancer. During menopause, ask your doctor to take an HPV culture at the time of your Pap smear. If it is negative for high-risk strains of the virus, and you have never had a problem with HPV or abnormal smears, Pap smears can be reduced to every two to three years—as long as you have a stable sex life (that is, a monogamous sex partner whom you trust.) If you have had a hysterectomy and no longer have a cervix, you do not need Pap smears. I still recommend yearly internal exams (or ultrasounds) to monitor your ovaries.
- To assess your heart disease risk factors, have your doctor order a thyroid screen, fasting lipid profile, CRP, homocysteine, and a diabetic screen with a HBA1C (hemoglobin A1C).
- All women (and their men friends) should have a colonoscopy by age fifty.

Is Estrogen Really Safe, Really?

Although I discussed hormone safety in chapter 3, here we are again. It's like that with my patients when the topic of estrogen comes up. Progesterone doesn't usually raise too many eyebrows, but the minute I mention estrogen I see the worry lines, literally. When estrogen support is needed, I have to address your fears all over again. And who can blame you. If you choose to use estrogen, you usually have to defend your decision to your friends, sisters, mother, and even other doctors. To help gain the confidence to defend your choice, understand some facts about estrogen.

Estrogen Facts

Estrogen is a creative force. It is stimulating to cells—that's its very nature. This effect is kept in check by the opposing effects of progesterone, a calming force. Critics of natural hormones are correct when they say that natural hormones carry risks. But if natural hormones are used safely and wisely, the risks can be minimized—and not using them is risky, too. Heart disease, dementia, bone loss, depression, urinary infections, and sexual dysfunction result from too little estrogen. There are two major risks of using any form of estrogen, natural or synthetic: excess blood clotting and excess cell stimulation leading to fibroids, cysts, and possibly cancer. So let's deal with the risks right up front.

Increased Blood Clotting

Blood clots are six times more likely to occur during pregnancy than at any other time in a woman's life. Control of blood clotting is normally carefully regulated by estrogen, progesterone, and clotting proteins made in your liver. During pregnancy, a woman's high levels of estrogen (particularly estriol) are balanced by equally high levels of progesterone, which naturally prevent excess clotting. Synthetic progesterone, medroxyprogesterone, does not act like natural progesterone to prevent clots. So always balance estrogen with natural progesterone to protect yourself from clotting.

It is also important to always use estrogen transdermally, never orally. Estrogen taken orally alters clotting proteins to promote further clotting. Our ovaries normally secrete hormones directly into our bloodstream, so the liver doesn't receive a high level of sex hormones. But hormones taken orally are absorbed through our gut and reach the liver immediately in high levels, which causes a rise in clotting proteins and predisposes to blood clots. Hormones given via the skin avoid these effects on the liver.

Increased Risks of Breast and Uterine Cancer

Once again, the problem is with synthetic hormones. Estrogen normally stimulates the cells that line the uterus and our breast cells, but it is normally balanced with natural progesterone to prevent overstimulation of these cells. Though synthetic progesterone, medroxyprogesterone (Provera), has been shown to reduce overgrowth of the uterine lining in response to estrogen, its effects are not the same on the breast. Provera increases the growth of breast cells and even promotes breast cancer. All studies using Provera and other synthetic progesterones show an increase in breast cancer over time. This is not true for natural progesterone. Natural progesterone taken orally, transdermally, or even vaginally, reduces the estrogen stimulation of the breast.

Using Natural Bioidentical Estrogen

There are many bioidentical estrogen products to choose from. Estradiol is available by prescription as a compounded or FDA-approved transdermal skin cream, lotion, gel, patch, vaginal cream, vaginal pellet, vaginal ring insert, and topical mist. I recommend using compounded skin lotion for the following reasons:

- Compounded products allow your hormones to be put in a paraben-free base.
- Compounded products can vary the concentration so that small amounts (around 1 ml or less) are needed.
- Using lotion is easier, faster, and less messy to apply.
- The most important reason: you are able to adjust the dose to your symptoms. This is essential during perimenopause, when your own hormone levels are changing so much. During menopause your needs will vary over time also. Compounding lets you use a minimum dose that's just right for you.

Using Compounded Lotions

Obtain a prescription from your doctor and get your hormones from a reputable compounding pharmacist who verifies concentrations and doesn't use parabens in the lotion base. For estradiol lotion I recommend a concentration of 1.0 mg/ml. This concentration avoids confusion when adjusting your dose or when you speak with your doctor because one ml is equal to one mg. Ask your pharmacist to dispense your lotion in a bottle with a syringe cap and to give you a syringe for accurate and adjustable dosing. (Some compounding pharmacies may dispense your estradiol in prefilled syringes, which can make varying your dose difficult.)

Some doctors may suggest using Biestrogen, a combination of estriol and estradiol. I don't usually recommend starting with this because if you are having symptoms or have had a hysterectomy you really need estradiol. Estriol is just too weak and won't control symptoms fully. Once you are settled on a stable estradiol dose, you can measure your estriol in a twenty-four-hour urine test. If it is too low (lower than 5 ug per twenty-four hours), add some estriol to the estradiol, creating Biestrogen. If this is necessary, I usually use 80 percent estradiol and 20 percent estriol. On occasion, I will use higher amounts of estriol, say if there is a history of breast cancer (discussed later). Never use triestrogen (estrone, estradiol, and estriol). Menopausal women produce excess estrones, some of which may be harmful, so it doesn't make sense to add more to your body.

Apply the lotion from your syringe to your inner and outer arm. Rub the lotion in well, for a full minute, so that all cream is absorbed. Your inner skin is thin and allows rapid absorption of the lotion; your outer arm has thicker skin that allows for a longer, delayed effect. Most lotions are fully absorbed into your body within one hour. For this reason I recommend using the lotion when you get up, even if you plan to exercise. Within one hour you should have fully absorbed your dose and you won't risk forgetting to apply it later.

Estrogen lotions should not be applied to the abdomen or breasts (as is often done with progesterone cream). You may want to alternate arms. Remember "Right at night" and "Left during the day." Alternating arms helps to avoid excess buildup of hormone in fat cells. Some doctors advise varying the sites to the inner or outer thighs, but I find that absorption there can be erratic. If you are confused, discuss this with your doctor. Your symptoms and levels will tell you how well you are absorbing your lotion. In general, don't use other lotions or creams on your arm at the same time.

Other Bioidentical Estrogen Options

There are now several FDA-approved estradiol gels, creams, patches, and, most recently, a mist spray. Unfortunately, these are fixed-dose products that are usually fixed too high to use in perimenopause and not high enough for menopause. They are, however, a step in the right direction and because of them we are now seeing more studies verifying the positive effects of transdermal estradiol, without the side effects of clotting.

Estrogel and its low-dose sister, Elestrin, are 0.06 percent estradiol gels. The former provides 0.75 mg of estradiol, the latter gives 0.5 mg per dose. Estrasorb is a cream (2.5 mg/gm in 1.74 gm pouches) that is poorly absorbed. For this reason it requires large doses (which are applied to the legs). Using Estrasorb is cumbersome, messy, and time-consuming. The recommended dose of two pouches (which is an awful lot of cream to rub in) requires three full minutes to apply. Now that doesn't sound like a lot of time, but trust me, it is an eternity on a busy, cold morning.

Though not perfect, I do feel that these topical products are a better alternative to estradiol patches. Patches vary from 0.025 to 0.1 mg and are changed one or two times per week, depending on the brand. The problems with patches are (1) they frequently cause skin irritation; (2) they often fall off—typically during warmer weather or with excess sweating (something menopausal women tend to do); and (3) it can be challenging to get the right dose. Some women cut the patches if the dose doesn't feel quite right, but patches won't work properly if they are cut. Having said this, some women like patches and use them happily.

Evamist, the first metered dose estradiol spray, was approved by the FDA in July 2007. Each spray delivers 1.5 mg of estradiol and takes two minutes to dry. Preliminary studies show that 13 percent of women using it developed nipple pain (too much estradiol). I expect there will be more topical sprays in lower doses in the future. The jury is still out on this one.

Vaginal Estrogen Preparations

The vagina is a world unto itself and vaginal estrogen preparations are often needed to protect that world—or at least to make it a more comfortable place. The cells that line your vagina and urethra are believed to be the most sensitive to low estrogen levels. A vaginal or urinary infection is often one of the first signs that your estradiol level is too low. If your estrogen levels are chronically low, you can develop atrophic vaginitis. It is estimated that 40 percent of postmenopausal women suffer from this. When it occurs, the cells that line your vagina shrink, or atrophy, causing your vaginal wall to thin and become dry. This may cause vaginal itching, burning, or bleeding; less intense orgasms; painful intercourse; urinary frequency (often disrupting sleep); or stress incontinence (loss of urine while coughing, laughing, or straining). When the vagina is too dry, bacteria and yeast become imbalanced, and chronic infections, irritation, and discharge can develop. If you have problems with recurrent urinary and/or vaginal infections, you need to balance your vaginal hormones in addition to correcting yeast and bacterial imbalance.

All forms of vaginal estrogen stimulate the cells lining the uterus. If you've had a hysterectomy and therefore don't have a uterus, there is of course no worry; but if you have a uterus, you must protect yourself by using progesterone. Always report any abnormal vaginal bleeding to your doctor. If this occurs, most physicians will recommend stopping or reducing the vaginal estrogen dose. Doctors may do an ultrasound to see how thick the lining of the uterus is or take a biopsy of your uterus (which can be done in an office visit). If your uterine lining is not too thick or the biopsy is normal, you can restart estrogen, but at a lower, less frequent dose. If you are using vaginal estradiol and have a bleeding problem, you should consider changing to the weaker estrogen, estriol. This works very well vaginally (see below).

Men should not be exposed to estrogen. Estriol is less of a threat to men than estradiol, but if you are having sexual relations, use vaginal estrogen during the day. If you must use it at night, have your partner wash his privates after intercourse.

Forms of Vaginal Estrogen

Vaginal estrogen is available by prescription as estradiol in vaginal pills, ring inserts, or creams. It can also be compounded as estradiol or estriol in a cream or vaginal pellet. Don't use forms of estrogen vaginally that are not natural bioidentical.

Estriol vaginal suppositories or cream is what I prefer to prescribe for my patients. Though estriol is a weaker estrogen than estradiol, it seems to be more effective vaginally, and it is safer to use, because it is less strong and less likely to overstimulate your uterine lining. Estriol is probably the best form to use vaginally if you have a history of fibroids or a tendency to spot or bleed with estradiol, and estriol may be safer for women with a history of breast cancer. I typically prescribe compounded estriol pellets in either a 1 mg or 2 mg dose (start with the lower dose first). Estriol can also be compounded into a vaginal cream, usually 1 or 2 mg/gm, which can be inserted with a vaginal dispenser.

Estradiol vaginal tablets or cream are available by prescription, as Estrace vaginal cream (0.01.percent) or Vagifem tablets (25 mcg of estradiol). These are useful for vaginal symptoms. Many women find the cream to be more soothing than the tablets. The tablets are less messy, but some women find them to be drying or irritating.

Vaginal ring inserts are favored by many women, as they are less messy and are effective for about three months, when they must be replaced. The vaginal ring, Femring, comes in two strengths of estradiol (0.05 mg and 0.10 mg per day) and can be used to treat vaginal symptoms as well as systemic symptoms such as hot flashes. Because its dose is so high, it should be used with natural progesterone. The Estring delivers less estradiol (0.075 mg/day) and is used to treat vaginal symptoms only. Vaginal inserts are usually well tolerated but they can fall out (rarely) when straining for a bowel movement, and they have been known to cause vaginal discomfort or irritation. Because the Femring delivers a higher dose, vaginal bleeding is more common with it than with the Estring.

Using Vaginal Estrogen

Use vaginal estradiol or vaginal estriol suppositories or creams the same way. Initially, use it every night for five to ten days to replenish all of the vaginal cells with estrogen. After this, use it only every two to three days. If it is used excessively, your uterine lining can become thickened. If this happens, you will have abnormal bleeding. Long-term overuse of vaginal estrogen can place you at risk for hyperplasia or (rarely) uterine cancer, so always discuss excessive or unusual bleeding with your doctor.

Estrogen Dosing

The best dose for estrogen is the one that alleviates your hot flashes, headaches, and mood changes, but doesn't cause breast tenderness, spotting, or irregular or excessive bleeding. Whether you are young, perimenopausal, or in the throes of menopause, it comes down to common sense and what feels right for you.

Doses vary depending on whether you are using a gel, cream, or spray. The base used in your compounding lotion can cause variations, too. Assuming that your progesterone dose is adequate, the following are signs that you need to adjust your estrogen dose:

- **Too much estrogen** will cause breast or nipple pain or swelling, irregular spotting or bleeding, excessive bleeding, headaches, irritability, anxiety, or insomnia.
- **Too little estrogen** will cause hot flashes, depression, insomnia, vaginal dryness, and urinary frequency.

I tell all women that they have estrogen meters inside them, their breasts. You will know almost immediately if you are using too much estrogen because your nipples and breasts tell you. If you develop tenderness, use a lower dose on the next application (reduce by 0.1 or 0.2 mg). Reducing usually works, but if you start having hot flashes or other low estrogen symptoms when you reduce, raise your progesterone, call your doctor, or check blood levels of your hormones to find out what's going on. You may not be absorbing your progesterone or not measuring your estrogen accurately, or your body may not be processing your hormones well (in which case I would use sitosterol or liver herbs).

If your estrogen lotion is applied correctly, your dose should last twelve hours. If you're having hot flashes toward the end of the day or night, check how well you are measuring and applying your lotion. You may not be applying it to the outer arm as well as you are applying it to the inner arm, so even though it may be absorbed well from your inner arm, it is not being absorbed well enough from your thicker outer skin to allow the dose to last the full twelve hours.

Always measure your lotion out each time, no matter how tempted you are to "guestimate." If you need to lower your dose, don't lower only one dose per day, lower both doses when using it twice daily. Sometimes women need less estrogen during the day, but if they lower the night dose they find themselves waking hot or sweaty. If this is happening, simply use a slightly bigger dose (0.1 or 0.2 mg more) at bedtime and a lower dose in the daytime. If you hate dosing twice daily, there are compounding pharmacies that make a once-daily estradiol gel, but I find that the twice-daily lotion works better.

If symptoms of low estrogen persist (hot flashes, headache, depression), increase the dose by 0.1 to 0.2 mg immediately and use the higher dose at the next application.

Cycling and Dosing Hormones

There is considerable debate and discussion about cycling hormones. In perimenopause there is no question that your hormones must be cycled but there is debate about what to do in menopause. Guess what? The answer is: do what feels best to you.

In Perimenopause

Stopping and starting estrogen will not disrupt your menstrual cycle or cause bleeding (unlike progesterone, which will cause you to bleed if it is suddenly stopped), so you can use estrogen any day of your cycle. Here are some general rules to follow:

During perimenopause estrogen is usually used on days 5 through 25 (day 1 is the first day of your period). Initially, you may feel best using it on days 1 through 25, especially if you are having menstrual headaches, depression, or fatigue. These symptoms should stop after a few days, once you are on the correct dose of estrogen. Most women feel better almost immediately.

For a cycle or two after you start, your menstrual symptoms, particularly menstrual headaches, may continue to be a problem. If so, use estradiol on days 1 to 25. These symptoms should stop altogether when you are well regulated. Once your menstrual symptoms stop, you can start taking hormonal breaks (use it on days 5 to 25). Stop it for a few days each month during your period (when all sex hormones are normally low). Anytime that you are off estrogen and you develop symptoms, go back on. Be prepared to change your dose according to how you feel. Remember, estrogen levels will vary day to day and cycle to cycle in perimenopause.

Add progesterone on days 15 to 25, as discussed in chapter 8. If you forget a progesterone dose or stop it too soon, expect to bleed or spot. That's what your body is supposed to do when progesterone levels suddenly drop.

Most perimenopausal women need very low doses of estradiol, typically only 0.1 to 0.4 mg, twice daily. If you miss a period, you are probably not on enough estradiol or your ovary was not producing enough to bleed that month. Simply determine when your period was due, and use this estimate as day 1. Restart your estradiol based on this date and add in progesterone two weeks later from this estimated day 1. This will maintain your progesterone cycle and keep your cycles regular. If you don't bleed again, then next cycle increase the estradiol and let your doctor know. Continue to estimate when your period was due and cycle accordingly. Keep in mind that you may skip three or four cycles in the later stages of perimenopause. As long as you are feeling well and following a cycle with your hormones, no matter. If you are confused or not feeling right, call your doctor. A blood test may be needed to determine if you are absorbing your estrogen or progesterone creams adequately.

In Menopause

Using hormones during menopause is easier than during perimenopause, because your estradiol levels are no longer fluctuating. You can cycle or you can take hormones continuously. Both are okay and it depends upon the individual. I generally prescribe progesterone every day with estradiol for my menopausal patients. Some doctors recommend cycling throughout menopause. A problem with this is that you are more likely to bleed, requiring an unnecessary biopsy or, worse, masking uterine hyperplasia or uterine cancer. Most of the women I meet don't want to think about cycling anymore, they've had enough. I have prescribed continuous use of natural estrogen and progesterone for my menopausal patients for years without serious problems. Discuss cycling with your doctor and see what works best for you.

Most menopausal women require 0.6 to 1.2 mg of estradiol twice daily. If hot flashes are severe you will probably need at least 0.8 mg doses. No matter what dose you start with, if you are having hot flashes, take a little more and increase the full dose at your next application. There is no reason to suffer for hours. Your tender breasts and other symptoms such as hot flashes will guide you. If your breasts are sore, you are on too much. If they are okay but you are having hot flashes, increase your dose. Always change doses gradually—by 0.1 or 0.2 mg at a time.

Once you have figured out the best dose for estrogen and progesterone, you can ask to have your hormones combined into one cream, which makes applications even easier. If you end up needing testosterone (discussed below), this can be added as well (another reason that I prefer compounding).

How Long?

Menopausal women often ask me how long they should stay on hormones. I advise using hormone support as long as you need to—as long as you have symptoms. Most women stop having symptoms by their sixtieth birthday, but we are all different. Over time, if your other hormones, such as thyroid, DHEA, cortisol, pregnenolone, and growth hormone, are balanced, you should need less estrogen and progesterone or possibly no sex hormones at all.

Studies, including the WHI study, have shown that using hormones in the first ten years of menopause (between the ages of fifty and fifty-nine) appears to reduce the risks of heart disease and plaque formation (hardening of the arteries). Age-guided studies can be misleading. What seems to be most important is the number of years from menopause. Some women enter menopause in their forties, others as late as their mid-fifties. It appears that using hormones in the first ten years of menopause is key to preventing bone disease, heart disease, probably dementia, and possibly Parkinson's disease.

Increased clotting risks have discouraged women from using hormones, particularly beyond age fifty-nine, but these studies used oral estrogen and synthetic progesterone, both known to increase clotting. European studies, including the ESTHER study published in 2006, showed no increased clotting when transdermal estrogen and natural progesterone were used. The age ranges in this study were forty-five to seventy years old (mean age 61.5 years).

So how safe are hormones after you hit sixty? Most doctors will tell you they are unsafe, but their logic is largely based on synthetic, oral estrogen and progestin studies. It is still unclear, but here is some of what we know:

- Once heart disease exists, starting hormone therapy does not appear to reverse it and, in fact, may make it more hazardous.
- All forms of hormone use (synthetic and natural) reduce bone loss and fractures.
- With regard to dementia, things are less clear because the studies used synthetic oral estrogen and synthetic progesterone. Despite this, these studies generally show that dementia improves if women have symptoms of menopause and use hormones within ten years of menopause. The WHI study examined older women (most were in their sixties and older) who had no symptoms of menopause and who were for the most part more than ten years away from menopause. Women who began synthetic hormones ten or more years after menopause appear to increase their risk of dementia.

So, here is what I recommend. Use natural hormones when you need them, early on in perimenopasue and menopause, and use them for at least ten years. Then reevaluate your need considering your health, risk factors, and symptoms. Do you have bone loss? What are your heart risk factors? Is there a family history of heart disease or stroke? No one answer will be right for all women. That is outdated thinking; we are not practicing McMedicine anymore.

Sheila Part 2: Menopause Begins

Remember Sheila from chapter 8? The woman who learned to take care of her PMS and other perimenopausal symptoms with progesterone? Well, when she turned forty-nine, she came to see me and reported, "Things are definitely different." Though her cycles were happening every twenty-eight days using progesterone, her bleeding lasted only two days. Her sex drive was "fine," and she was actually getting married for the first time at the age of fifty. We discussed the signs and symptoms of low estradiol so that she would know what to watch out for. Months later, she returned from her honeymoon reporting skipped periods, some vaginal dryness, and a urinary infection, something that had never been a problem. She also noted that her sex drive was lower and her memory was failing for many names and phone numbers. In addition, she had developed menstrual cramping in the first day or two of her period, another new symptom. She was also starting to feel hot at night and was not sleeping well.

So we discussed estrogen. I went through all of the studies and charts. She agreed to try it: "Anything to feel balanced again." I prescribed estradiol lotion (1.0 mg/ml) and told her to apply 0.5 ml twice daily, to her inner and outer arms, alternately, on days 1 to 25 of her cycle. I told her to continue to cycle in progesterone on days 15 to 25, and that if she was too hot, she should increase the dose of estradiol to 0.6 ml. I cautioned her that if her breasts were sore or she spotted, she should lower the estradiol dose by one-half and call me. I also gave her a calendar to help her figure out when to start and stop her creams, explaining that if her cycle didn't come, use the date that it was due as day 1 and restart progesterone two weeks later. I told her that if her vaginal dryness didn't get better, she could add an estriol (1 mg) vaginal suppository to make intercourse more comfortable and prevent any further urinary infections. Her symptoms improved using 0.6 ml estradiol twice daily with cycled progesterone; she didn't need vaginal estriol, at least for the time being.

Wendy: Perimenopause to Menopause

When I met Wendy she was fifty-three years old and had been on oral contraceptives for four years to control irregular periods. She used to enjoy normal energy, but in the past year she had become progressively less energetic and was especially tired in the afternoon between 2 and 4 p.m. Her usual upbeat mood had left her. She was often sick and frequently took antibiotics for recurrent sinus infections. Her periods had always been headache-free, but now she was getting headaches in the days before her period, and her breasts were tender for a full week before she bled. She was experiencing dry eyes and vaginal dryness. Her sleep was okay, but she didn't feel refreshed when she woke up in the morning. She had been diagnosed with osteopenia, for which she was doing push-ups.

She was reluctant to change her birth control pills, but she was eager to start an adrenal extract to improve her energy while we waited for her lab results. Within days on the adrenal support, her mood improved and she had better energy, but she was still not back to normal. She still felt tired, particularly when she was stressed.

Her blood tests showed a high level of sex hormone binding globulin (SHBG), and her twenty-four-hour urine test, which measures free, unbound hormones, showed a low level of cortisol, very low DHEA, and low testosterone. Blood tests also revealed that her DHEA level was very low, as was her estradiol level. I explained to her that taking an oral contraceptive had caused her liver to make extra SHBG which, in addition to binding her estradiol (so it wouldn't work) was binding other hormones, including cortisol and testosterone.

She agreed to stop her oral contraceptive and start using transdermal estradiol and progesterone. I explained to her that whenever you switch from oral contraceptives to natural hormones, you should complete your cycle of oral contraceptives and start your estrogen on what would have been the first day of another cycle of pills to avoid disrupting your own hormone rhythms. I told her that it would take a few months for her SHBG to return to normal, so she would probably need more estradiol and adrenal support initially. I prescribed 0.8 mg of estradiol twice daily, with instructions to reduce her dose if she developed any breast tenderness. I also started her on progesterone transdermal skin lotion (125 mg twice daily, starting on day 15 of her cycle, for ten days) and DHEA (10 mg daily). I increased her adrenal extract and told her to take it when her body normally produced it, in the morning, with a lower dose at noon.

She developed breast tenderness, but she knew to reduce her estradiol dose and found that she only needed 0.2 ml twice daily. She continued the progesterone as prescribed. Her cycles came regularly every twenty-eight days, just as they had on the birth control pills, but she no longer had mood problems, fatigue, headaches, or vaginal or eye dryness. She also stopped getting frequent colds. After a few months, she gradually stopped the DHEA and used the adrenal extract every few days, when she felt run-down or tired.

After a year of treatment, she felt so good that she wasn't sure she needed any support, so she stopped everything to see what would happen. She did okay initially, but after a few weeks she noticed that her sleep had become less solid. A year later off the hormones, she also developed some cramping with her periods, along with very dry eyes, and her bone density fell further, so she restarted estradiol and progesterone.

Wendy continued on this regimen for another two years. As she approached her fifty-fifth birthday, her cycles became more erratic (she began skipping periods) and I told her to use progesterone every day if she started to miss periods routinely. By age fifty-seven, her periods ended even though she continued on cycled hormones. At that time, she decided to continue using a low dose of estradiol and progesterone daily, for bone health (which had improved) and to support her mood and sleep. Currently, she is on a low dose of estradiol (0.5 mg twice daily) and progesterone cream (125 mg twice daily), with some Panax ginseng and a low dose of DHEA to support her adrenal glands and bones, and testosterone (2.5 mg/day), to help her feel more balanced.

Hormones after Hysterectomy

It is estimated that 22 million women living in the United States have had some or all of their female organs removed. Of the 617,000 women who underwent hysterectomies in 2004, 73 percent had both ovaries removed. One-third of all women can expect to have a hysterectomy (removal of the uterus and sometimes one or both ovaries) by the age of sixty.

Our uterus is a sex organ and an important support for our bladder and bowels. Even if ovaries are left intact, the blood flow to the ovaries is affected and most women become menopausal nearly four years earlier than expected. Many women who experience uterine orgasms lose that ability after a hysterectomy. An even greater loss of sexual well-being may be felt if both ovaries are removed.

Removing a woman's ovaries, though often necessary, is not to be undertaken lightly. We are often led to believe that our ovaries don't do too much once we hit menopause, but after menopause our ovaries continue to make testosterone and dozens of other hormones, many of which are still not fully understood. I always advise women to keep their ovaries if possible. Premenopausal women undergoing ovarian hysterectomy have an increased risk of osteoporosis and death from heart disease. A 2005 study published in the *American Journal of Obstetrics and Gynecology* reported that for women who had their ovaries removed between the ages of fifty and fifty-four, the likelihood of reaching their eightieth birthday was reduced by 9 percent.

It is important to remember that even if you no longer have a uterus, you still need to use natural progesterone if you are using estrogen. Studies have shown that perimenopausal women who are deficient in progesterone have a greater risk of breast cancer. If you are perimenopausal, using hormones after a hysterectomy can be tricky. Without your monthly bleed it can be difficult to know just when to cycle your progesterone. But using it will reduce breast pain, along with the risk of breast cancer, bone loss, and even clotting problems associated with unopposed estrogen. Most women can still feel their cycles after a hysterectomy and can estimate when to cycle progesterone. You could use progesterone continuously, but for some women that doesn't always work. See the example below.

Patty: Hormones after Hysterectomy

Patty was forty-nine when she remarried and became stepmother to two young children. She had raised her own three children single-handedly, but she was prepared to do it all again. At the age of forty-five, she'd had a hysterectomy because of heavy persistent uterine bleeding from a large fibroid. No one ever discussed hormones with her. She had chosen to keep her ovaries, so she thought she was okay.

About a year after her hysterectomy, she developed hypertension and was started on a diuretic. She also developed very tender, swollen breasts and was diagnosed with fibrocystic breast disease. Her breasts were sore and swollen for nearly two weeks every month. When I met her at the age of forty-nine she was a bit more tired, but she was, "after all, running after two small children and adjusting to her new life." She used to sleep soundly, but now she was having insomnia most nights and feeling irritable and discouraged with things. Her sex drive was not what it should be, and she suffered from recurrent urinary infections.

On examination, her breasts were tender and lumpy, and her abdomen was bloated and distended. Blood tests showed a normal estradiol level, and her FSH and LH indicated that she was not yet menopausal. Her magnesium, calcium, and potassium were in the very lowest ranges of normal, as was her DHEA. Her cortisol was okay, but her aldosterone was high.

I started her on oral progesterone at bedtime, in addition to some potassium aspartate and a calcium/magnesium supplement. We decided to see what progesterone alone would do before adding any DHEA. I compounded 100 mg progesterone and told her to start with one pill (100 mg) at bedtime to see how she would react to it, and increase to 200 mg at bedtime if things felt okay. I explained that she should try to cycle her progesterone, starting it as soon as she detected any breast tenderness or worsening insomnia and use it for ten days.

She slept better using one, so she increased it to two. She was so thankful to sleep better, and her breast pain improved almost immediately. She continued the progesterone every day, since she felt so great. One day she called, saying that she thought the progesterone was making her depressed. She couldn't stop crying. When I asked how she was cycling the progesterone, she said that she had felt so good on it that she never stopped it. She had been on the progesterone for nearly twenty days. I explained that she was out of sync with her cycling estrogen. She stopped the progesterone, and immediately her mood lifted. She waited until she thought her breasts were fuller and she believed she had ovulated. Sure enough, some irritability resurfaced, so she restarted the progesterone. As expected, her mood improved and she slept well. This time she remembered to write on her calendar a reminder to stop her progesterone in ten days. She was amazed at how her breasts were no longer sore or lumpy on the progesterone, and she has continued to cycle progesterone for ten days every month. She feels balanced and in control, despite having had a hysterectomy.

Mary: Estrogen and Progesterone after Hysterectomy

When I met Mary, she was a forty-five-year-old school administrator with two grown children. She told me that uncontrollable bleeding from uterine fibroids had caused her to have a hysterectomy at age thirty-six. Her ovaries were left in. She felt fine after the surgery except for the onset of some migraines and irritable bowel syndrome.

By the time she turned forty-four, things started to fall apart. Hot flashes woke her in the middle of the night, and she had no energy, suffered from depression, and was having trouble remembering everyday things like phone numbers and people's names. Sex wasn't fun anymore. "I felt as dry as sandpaper," she reported. Her doctor prescribed synthetic estrogen, Premarin, but not progesterone since she didn't have a uterus.

Premarin improved her hot flashes and vaginal dryness, but her headaches persisted and eventually worsened. After about four months her sleep became light and fitful, interrupted by frequent trips to the bathroom to urinate. She still had no energy, and her irritable bowel symptoms grew worse. Media reports about Premarin began to trouble her. It seemed that every day she read something in the newspaper about its possible links to dementia and breast cancer. She was scared to stay on it.

I recommended that Mary switch from synthetic oral hormone replacement to bioidentical natural hormones. Instead of Premarin, she used natural estradiol and progesterone skin lotions. To support her adrenals, she took an adrenal extract and pregnenolone.

Mary did well on her new regimen. Her energy bounced back almost immediately. Initially she had some hot flashes, but increasing the estradiol lotion fixed that. Her thyroid blood test, though within normal range, was on the low side of normal, so I put her on a low dose of active thyroid hormone. Her irritable bowel symptoms improved and her migraines stopped. Natural cortisol in a very low dose (2.5 to 5mg/day) was added three months later for a short time (three to four months) to address fatigue. She is now on a very low dose of estradiol and progesterone lotion and no longer needs active thyroid or adrenal supports. She reports that she is sleeping normally with good energy—as she describes it, "Like I used to feel."

Beyond Breast Cancer

The good news about breast cancer is that both the number of new cases and the number of deaths from breast cancer have been on the decline since 2000. This decline preceded the publication of the WHI study results, so clearly the reduced hormone use generated by that study was not solely responsible. The more probable reason for this decline is that women are being diagnosed earlier, with a more treatable disease. In particular, breast MRIs for suspicious or especially dense mammograms and advancements in needle biopsies have allowed pre-cancerous lesions (hyperplasia and cancer in situ) and early cancers to be detected, and treatments have become more effective. The fact remains that most women who develop breast cancer will die from heart disease and suffer from menopausal symptoms like any other woman.

So what should you do if you are a woman who has beaten breast cancer? To begin with, you need to learn why you developed cancer and what you can do to prevent its recurrence in the future. Some oncologists and cancer surgeons don't see this as their job. Once you've had the cancerous mass removed and undergone radiation or chemotherapy, you are proclaimed "cancer-free" and sent back out into the world with a congratulatory handshake and blessings of good luck. After such visits, you are left to your own devices to figure out when or if cancer will strike again, without a clue as to what you can do to prevent it.

You need to be proactive. There are things you can do to better understand your cancer risks, and there are many reliable studies showing that some forms of estrogen can be used safely to treat menopausal symptoms after cancer.

Other Treatments for Menopausal Symptoms

Hormones are not for everyone, particularly women with a past history of breast cancer, so here are a few alternatives to make life feel better if you are suffering.

Black cohosh (*cimicifuga racemosa*) was originally used by Native Americans to treat menstrual cramps and menopausal symptoms. Multiple studies have shown that black cohosh can effectively alleviate hot flashes, and this herb is now routinely prescribed to treat hot flashes. Concerns for its use by women with a history of breast cancer appear to be unfounded. A 2007 study showed that there was no increase in mammogram density or endometrial biopsies after six months of use. Other studies using breast cancer cells (with estrogen-postive receptors) showed that there was no stimulation of the receptors. This study also showed that Tamoxifen (a drug used in women at risk for breast cancer or to prevent breast cancer recurrence) effects were increased, not decreased. A Japanese study indicates that black cohosh inhibits breast cancer cells.

Black cohosh is available in tinctures, tablets, and capsules. The usual dose is 40 to 80 mg daily (2 to 4 ml of tincture, three times daily), but be aware that since its full effects may not be felt for two to three weeks, it is not much help if you need immediate relief. It works best over the long term. Because most studies of black cohosh lasted only six months, that is the recommended duration for its use, but I have prescribed it longer without ill effects.

Vitamin E (800 mg/day) with **evening primrose oil** (4000 mg/day) has been shown to be helpful for hot flashes.

Targeted amino acid therapies to support serotonin and epinephrine levels can dramatically help with sleep, mood, and hot flashes.

Chinese herbal products, primarily "yin tonics," are very effective and have been used for centuries to treat menopausal symptoms including hot flashes, insomnia, and depression. Such treatments can be more effective when coupled with acupunture.

Vaginal vitamin E suppositories can be compounded and work well for vaginal dryness. A New Zealand product made from kiwi fruit, marketed as "Sylk," is chemical-free, and is a helpful sexual lubricant.

Supplements and Lifestyle after Breast Cancer

Here are some things to consider doing to improve your odds against breast cancer recurrence:

- Read chapters 3 and 4 to understand how cancer might have formed in you and how environment plays a role.
- Use of antioxidants is controversial during cancer treatments but after treatments are finished, you should rotate antioxidants as discussed in chapter 4.
- Eat a diet with plenty of fresh fruits and cruciferous vegetables. Avoid foods containing pesticides and other artificial chemicals or hormones.
- Avoid paraben-containing deodorants and body lotions.
- Limit your alcohol intake to a maximum of two or three drinks per week.
- Evaluate your genetic SNP to determine if inherited problems with estrogen metabolism are present.
- Methylation is essential for good estrogen metabolism. Evaluate your methylation abilities by measuring homocysteine in the blood and methylmalonic acid levels in the urine (offered by specialty labs). You may need vitamin B_6, or methylated folic acid and B_{12} if these are abnormal.
- Use I-3-C (400 mg/day) in addition to DIM, sitosterol, and ground flaxseeds to help metabolize estrogens more safely.
- Have your stool tested for an excess of glucuronidase, which is produced by bacteria in your gut. If your stool glucuronidase is high, improve your gut bacteria with herbs and probiotics and use calcium-d-glucarate to lower glucuronidase.
- Measure your heavy metal levels with a twenty-four-hour urine test. Mercury, lead, and other toxic metals will lower your body's antioxidant resources and make you prone to producing cancer causing quinones.
- Be sure that your thyroid function and iodine levels are optimal (see chapter 10).
- Maintain a normal weight. Exercise regularly and limit your intake of animal fats (for example, limit red meat to one to two

servings each week and substitute natural omega-3 spreads for butter).

Hormone Use after Breast Cancer

Women who have a history of breast cancer and decide to become pregnant do not appear to increase their risk of recurrence. Nine independent studies have shown that women with a history of breast cancer who use hormones have a better quality of life, no increase in recurrence of breast cancer, and no reduction in their life expectancy. One of the largest of these studies, performed in Australia, followed more than a thousand women from 1969 to 1999. This study reported that women who regularly used hormones had a reduced risk of death from breast cancer and a reduced risk of recurrence.

These results may seem surprising, but because some forms of estrogen (estriol and 2-methoxyestrone) have been shown to prevent breast cancer cell growth, there may be a true benefit from using estrogen, particularly estriol or supplements that increase 2-methoxyestrone levels. The decision must be made individually, between you and your doctor. But there are some things you can do to improve your odds and maintain the good quality of your life. In addition to the tips discussed above, consider the following points if you decide to use hormones:

- Don't use medroxyprogesterone (Provera) or other synthetic progesterone. Numerous studies, including the WHI study, have shown increased breast cancer with its use.
- Use only transdermal estrogen. If you decide to use it, consider using a combination of estriol and estradiol (some women opt to use only estriol). Studies show that women are more likely to get cancer when estriol is deficient.
- Use natural progesterone to prevent clotting and overstimulation of cells in the breast and uterus. Natural progesterone has never been shown to be carcinogenic.
- Monitor estrogen metabolites. Do this only if you are using estrogen, because results are not useful or reliable if your estrogen levels are very low.

Testosterone in Women

Testosterone builds bone, muscles, stamina, and confidence. It strengthens and moisturizes your skin and can help you lose weight. It definitely improves your sex drive and orgasmic ability. There are reasons I saved this for last: (1) I almost never prescribe it during perimenopause; (2) I never prescribe it without estradiol to balance it, and (3) it won't bolster a woman's sex drive like it will a man's. For these reasons, testosterone is the first sex hormone I offer men and usually the last hormone I offer women. But it is important, and I do use it frequently in women. I think of testosterone as the icing on the cake. Estrogen makes the cake, but testosterone makes it that much more delicious.

When you were a young woman, most of your testosterone came from your ovaries, but as early as your mid-thirties and early forties, your ovarian testosterone levels fell by about 50 percent. When you enter menopause, the fall stops. Testosterone is also made in your fat and skin from an important adrenal hormone, DHEA (dehydroepiandrosterone) or DHEA-S (dehydroepiandrosterone sulfate). In this way our adrenal glands continue to support our estrogen and testosterone as we age. Testosterone produced in our fat is important for building and preserving our bones, which explains why thin women are more prone to bone loss. Similarly, women with ovarian hysterectomies are especially prone to bone loss. But bone loss isn't the only problem associated with low testosterone in women.

Symptoms of Low Testosterone

How do you know if you need testosterone? If your bones and muscles are dwindling, your HDL is low, your sex drive is not what it used to be, you can no longer achieve orgasm, or your self-confidence is low, then you probably need testosterone support. Other symptoms include weight gain, especially around the belly, and failing memory. There are testosterone receptors in the brain, and studies have shown that women with memory loss show greater improvement when using estrogen with testosterone, instead of estrogen alone. If any of this sounds like you, ask your doctor to measure your testosterone level (remember to measure a free and a total level).

Testosterone Converts into Estrogen

Most people don't realize that testosterone converts into estrogen; in fact, without testosterone, women can't make estrogen. Even men convert testosterone into estrogen. It is part of their aging process. Look around and you will see older men growing breasts and becoming less competitive.

Testosterone conversion into estrogen is generally a good thing for women, but for men it is potentially harmful and one reason I caution women about exposing their men to estrogen, vaginally or systemically. Excess estrogen in men predisposes them to prostate and heart disease. The same problems of poor estrogen metabolism that predispose women to breast cancer also predispose men to prostate cancer. For this reason I always ask my patients about prostate cancer in their relatives. If they had several family members with prostate cancer, I may recommend doing genetic testing, and I certainly will monitor their estrogen metabolites closely. Just as diets high in flax, antioxidants, and cruciferous vegetables help to prevent breast cancer in women, such diets and nutrients can help to prevent prostate cancer in men.

Balancing Testosterone and Estrogen

Because most women make testosterone from their adrenal hormone, DHEA, I usually restore DHEA levels first to see if that will take care of low testosterone symptoms. If that doesn't work, then I supplement with testosterone. If you use testosterone, you must use it with estrogen. Estrogen and testosterone balance is needed for testosterone to be effective and to avoid side effects. The testosterone receptors in your brain actually depend on estradiol, so if your estrogen is low, you probably won't feel any better on testosterone. During menopause, you have a relative excess of testosterone compared with estrogen, which can have masculinizing effects. Hair may start growing on your chin while the hair on your head is thinning. You may notice more pimples, or even suffer from acne. Estrogen balances testosterone.

Measuring Testosterone

Unlike men, who have high testosterone levels in the early morning (hence their morning erections), women tend to produce testosterone evenly throughout the day. There is a cyclic variation, however, with the lowest production of testosterone during the week of the period (when all sex hormones, including estrogen and progesterone, are at their lowest). For this reason, if you are cycling, it is best to measure testosterone after day 7 of your cycle. Testosterone levels peak when you ovulate (nature's way of ensuring that you are most interested in sex during your most fertile time), so a mid-cycle level is going to be the highest of the month. Testosterone levels begin to fall gradually during early perimenopause, and they stay at about 50 percent of premenopausal levels for the rest of your life. Menopausal women can measure levels any time of day or any day of the month, because there is no longer any variation. When measuring testosterone, I always monitor DHEA-S levels, too.

Testosterone can be measured from your blood, urine, or saliva. Whatever test you choose, you must measure a "free level" (free testosterone) because testosterone travels in the body largely bound to the binding protein SHBG. This explains why women taking birth control pills or oral hormones (which cause a high level of SHBG) tend to have very low levels of free testosterone. Low testosterone explains why many women using oral contraceptives or oral estrogen experience a gradual decline in their sex drive over time and have a tendency to gain weight. Other causes of low testosterone are adrenal fatigue, pelvic surgery, traumatic childbirth, depression, excessively low-fat diets, and some medications, most notably lipid-lowering statin medications.

Testosterone Side Effects

Most women are frightened by the thought of using what is reputed to be an exclusively male hormone for fear of turning into an oversized, hairy, argumentative beast. But when used correctly, balanced with estrogen and progesterone, testosterone support can make you feel sexier and stronger than ever. On too much you could become overly opinionated, but you will not necessarily go on a rampage. Hair loss is the main reason that women stop using testosterone. Why? There is a protein or enzyme, known as reductase, which is found primarily on the skin, particularly in hairy areas, that converts testosterone into DHT, dihydrotestosterone. DHT, not testosterone, causes hair loss from the head and oily pimples and increases hair on the face and body.

These DHT effects are the major side effects of testosterone.

There are some things that you can do to limit DHT production. Progesterone, zinc (50 mg/day), and saw palmetto (320 mg/day) all reduce reductase activity and can prevent hair loss. Using enough estrogen to balance your testosterone also helps to preserve your locks.

Hair Loss 101

Hair loss is not just a problem for women using testosterone, it is a huge problem for many. At least one-half of all women in the United States, by the time they reach the age of fifty, have some problem with hair loss. Just look around the supermarket at all of the dwindling scalps. Most women suffer hair loss during perimenopause and menopause. At this age, most hair issues are due to thyroid problems (see chapter 10), estradiol deficiency, or a relative excess of testosterone.

There are different types of hair loss problems depending on your race, diet, hormones, and stress levels.

> **Shedding** (telogen effluvium) is when hair is lost from the entire scalp. With shedding, your hair is lost when you comb, brush, or wash your hair. Shedding hair can be caused by thyroid problems (too little or too much), medications, poor nutrition, yeast imbalance, or hormone imbalance. Any physical stress (surgery, illness, rapid change in weight) or emotional stress can cause hair loss. Usually, shedding hair loss will be noticeable around two to three months after the stress begins because it takes this long for hair to grow up your hair shaft.
>
> Other causes of shedding are high doses of vitamin A, blood pressure medications, certain antidepressants, gout medications, birth control pills, and low iron or zinc. The treatment for shedding is hormone support (estradiol and progesterone transdermal lotion), B vitamins (B_6 100 mg/day or B complex 100 mg/day), and high doses of biotin (15 to 25 mg/day). Shedding can be a problem after delivering a baby (due to low iron or hormones, lack of sleep, and low nutrients from the body's stress of breast-feeding). When shedding occurs during perimenopause or menopause, it is usually from a combination of poor sleep, low estrogen, and excessive dieting.

Female pattern hair loss (anagen effluvium) is common among menopausal women and is most common in forty- to fifty-something women when there is an imbalance of female and male hormones. This type of hair loss may be associated with using testosterone, but it can also be inherited. That is, you inherit an excessively active reductase enzyme with a tendency to produce more DHT from testosterone (or more androstanedione from DHEA). You know who you are. You are the passionate (DHT heightens sex drive), sexy women prone to excess body and facial hair. Hair is lost on the top of the scalp, rather than throughout, as with shedding. Hair becomes finer, as the hairs actually become smaller. Usually women notice that their ponytails are less thick or the part in the middle of their head is wider.

Treating Hair-Loss Problems

This topic could fill another book, and there are certainly plenty of books that deal exclusively with this. First, you want to test for the possible causes and then start treating the problem. Consider the following:

- Check DHT and androstanedione levels (male hormone metabolites)
- Check for iron deficiency: CBC, ferritin (iron stores)
- Measure RBC minerals or RBC magnesium and zinc
- Exclude hyper- or hypothyroid with blood tests TSH, free T3, and free T4 (thyroid tests)
- Measure levels of estradiol and progesterone (days 19 to 21 or any time you are using support)
- Exclude chronic yeast problems by measuring candida immune complexes and antibodies

Correct any problems discovered from your blood tests. If your male hormone metabolites are high (male pattern balding) or no cause for your hair loss is found, use the supplements listed below. Remember that it takes about two months for hair to grow up a follicle to your scalp, so expect to see improvement in two to three months.

- Take biotin, 15 to 30 mg daily.

- Take zinc, 50 mg daily.
- Take saw palmetto, 320 mg daily.

If your hair growth gets better but is not ideal, add the Chinese herbal blend Shou Wu Wan (also known as He Shou Wu or Shou Wu Pian). It is a single herb or a blend of herbs used for centuries, and it works. It is available on my Web site and in most Chinese herbal stores.

Excess Testosterone

Oily skin, oily hair, and pimples are usually the first signs of too much testosterone. Because testosterone converts into estrogen, too much testosterone can feel like too much estrogen and you may develop breast tenderness and swelling or even vaginal bleeding. Mood changes on too much testosterone are not what you might imagine. Rather than becoming violent or angry, you have excess confidence and can start to feel bossy, or overly authoritative.

Using Testosterone

Testosterone is the only hormone labeled by the FDA as a controlled substance because of its potential for abuse, most commonly by body-builders and athletes. It is now available for women by skin lotion, gel, injection, patch, and orally. For women I prescribe only skin lotions, but rarely some doctors prefer injections, typically for women with bone loss who cannot tolerate transdermal lotions.

> **Compounded transdermal testosterone** lotion is typically what I prescribe. The dose in women is variable; some women can use 5 mg without a problem and others cannot tolerate anything more than 1 mg. I usually prescribe 5 mg per ml and ask my patients to start with 0.2 ml (or 1 mg) per day and increase or decrease as needed. Because of side effects, I rarely use more than 5 mg per day. Because some women find it stimulating, testosterone is usu-ally used once daily, in the morning. It should be applied to a hair-less area (to limit reductase conversion of testosterone into its

hair-losing metabolite, DHT). I recommend applying the lotion to the outer thighs or inner arm. You must avoid getting testosterone on your face or chest because it will cause hair growth, and you must avoid getting it directly on your breasts because it converts into estrogen.

Transdermal patches and gel are now available by prescription. The patches come in doses of 2.5 mg or 5.0 mg, which is often too high for women. Androgel is marketed for men (in a 1 percent concentration). The smallest-size packets are 2.5 gm, which provides 25 mg of testosterone (much too high for women). Some doctors have women use one-fifth of a packet (5 mg) every other day, but I feel it is much easier and safer to have a compounding pharmacist prepare a less concentrated lotion.

Clitoral or vulvar testosterone can be compounded and can be particularly helpful if there is chronic vulvar irritation that won't improve with topical estrogen. Some few women find that vaginal testosterone cream heightens sexual arousal.

Oral testosterone should never be used because it can lead to liver disease or liver tumors. Giving testosterone through the skin (transdermally), by injection, or under the tongue (sublingually) avoids harm to the liver.

Conclusion

- Use transdermal estradiol and progesterone when needed during perimenopause and the first ten years of menopause.
- Use bioidentical estradiol transdermally and once you are on a stable, effective dose, do a twenty-four-hour urine test to determine if you need to add estriol and to monitor how safely estrogen is metabolizing in you.
- Monitor your estrogen metabolites in a twenty-four-hour urine text every year to ensure that you are not making too much 16-OH estrone or 4-OH estrone and that you are making enough 2-methoxyestrone.

- Use natural bioidentical progesterone orally or transdermally to balance your estrogen, even if you had a hysterectomy.
- Add vaginal estrogen if you need to (estriol may be the best form to use to avoid overstimulating the uterine lining).
- If you need to add testosterone, always use it with estrogen and progesterone to limit its side effects.
- If you experience hair loss or pimples using testosterone, lower the dose, and measure your DHT. Using saw palmetto (320 mg/day) and zinc (50 mg/day) can help reduce hair loss with it, especially if your DHT is too high.

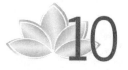

10

Adrenal and Thyroid Hormones

I f you have balanced your estrogen and progesterone, you may be feeling on top of the world. At least your hot flashes should have stopped, your cycles should be more tolerable, PMS and headaches should be gone or doing better, and sleep, if not good, should be deeper and more restful. You should be feeling more confident and back on your mark. So you're done, right? Wrong. How did your sex hormones get so out of balance? And what are you going to do about it? You could continue to use sex hormones to alleviate your symptoms, or you can delve deeper and learn how to get your body to produce more sex hormones on its own. You could take a hard look at your thyroid and adrenal glands.

Thyroid glands work closely with all of our glands, particularly our adrenals. Thyroid and adrenal glands are vital for the normal function of all of our sex hormones and affect our weight, energy, mood, bowels, sugar levels, muscles, and immune function. They maintain our energy and stamina, particularly as we age. This chapter will introduce you to these glands: what they do when they're working right, how to recognize when they're not, and how to support them in the short run and over the long term.

Adrenal and Thyroid Problems Are Common

Adrenal and thyroid deficiencies are common, but often go unrecognized. These deficiencies tend to occur during perimenopause and menopause, when we need all of the hormone support we can get. New patients often ask, "If I was meant to have sex hormones as I age, wouldn't I make them naturally?" The answer is yes, we are meant to produce sex hormones on our own as we age. That's where the adrenal glands fit in. Our adrenal glands, which lie on top of our kidneys, are well known for producing our stress hormones, cortisol and adrenaline. In addition, they also produce hormones that convert into the sex hormones progesterone, estrogen, and testosterone.

When our ovaries start to wind down during perimenopause, our adrenal glands, which had been comfortably pumping out stress hormones, are suddenly saddled with double duty—now producing sex hormones and stress hormones. When our adrenals tire, we tire easily, gain weight, are susceptible to colds, and become easily irritated.

Adrenal deficiency is so common that it has been dubbed The Twenty-First-Century Syndrome. Although growing awareness of this deficiency is relatively new to the West, adrenal fatigue has been known for centuries in China, where traditional treatments emphasize supporting the kidney to improve energy and sex drive. In China, middle-aged women routinely take herbs such as ginseng and licorice, which are important adrenal adaptogens, or adrenal supports. Here in the United States people haven't yet grasped the benefits of adpatogens, and we tend to self-medicate our low adrenals (and low thyroids) with caffeine, chocolate, stimulants, and diet pills. These only worsen our problems. It is no surprise that coffee shops have sprung up on every corner, and we are growing fatter as a nation. We are becoming a country of hormonally challenged individuals, running on unbalanced hormones and indulging ourselves in the wrong treatments.

But treating adrenal glands is not enough. Adrenal glands work closely with the thyroid. Our thyroid glands help our cells produce energy. Without enough thyroid hormones we feel, look, and act sluggish. Centuries ago, Chinese physicians recognized that these glands work together even though they are not located anywhere near each other (our thyroid gland wraps around the Adam's apple in our neck, and our adrenals lie atop our kidneys in our back). Western science is slowly catching up to this Chinese view, and it is now known that both adrenaline and thyroid hormones are made from the same amino acid, tyrosine. It is also known that if our adrenaline is low, our body will produce more thyroid hormone, and that too much cortisol will lower our thyroid hormones, and so on. Chinese medicine describes low thyroid symptoms as "kidney yang deficiency" and adrenal deficiency as "kidney yin deficiency." When these yin and yang glands are well balanced, they provide us with energy and stamina, and they support all of our other hormones.

So here are your next steps: (1) Understand how the adrenal and thyroid glands work together. (2) Recognize the symptoms of adrenal fatigue and thyroid imbalance. (3) Measure the hormones produced by these glands. (4) Learn how to support the adrenal and thyroid glands with natural hormones, herbs, and vitamins so that they can support your stress and sex hormones as you age.

How Our Adrenals and Thyroid Work Together

There are three major substances that give you your get-up-and-go: (1) thyroid hormone; (2) cortisol; and (3) adrenaline (epinephrine). If one of these three is low, the others rise to fill the gap. So if your thyroid hormone is low, your adrenal glands will increase production of adrenaline and other adrenal hormones, which may make you feel edgy or irritable and can raise your blood pressure. These symptoms are common in individuals with low thyroid function. Over time, this increased hormone production can be exhausting to the adrenal glands and they will sputter out. Similarly, if your cortisol is low, your thyroid will produce more thyroid hormone to compensate. In almost all cases of low cortisol and/or low thyroid, there is a raised adrenaline, or noradrenaline (the precursor to adrenaline) level, which can cause palpitations and anxiety and make you feel like you are running on fumes. Over time, however, even adrenaline can fall, and then most adrenal hormones will be low, too. This is the case with many chronic fatigue patients I see. They have lost adrenal support and often have a thyroid issue as well. Now, I am not saying this was the cause of their underlying fatigue, but adrenal and thyroid imbalance are often part of the problem.

Thyroid hormones support our ordinary day-to-day life needs. They regulate our body temperature, heart rate, how we burn fats, and how our nerves and muscles react. Our adrenals, on the other hand, handle the emergencies. Adrenaline, cortisol, and aldosterone enable us to cope with urgent needs—that is, to do battle. Though most of us are no longer fighting wild beasts or crossing swords in our daily lives, we are overworking, double-tasking, undersleeping, and in general running ourselves ragged dealing with everyday battles. Over time, this constant demand takes a toll, and our adrenal reserves fall. When this happens, it is difficult to handle stress. We reach for alcohol to settle our nerves or take pills to calm our moods and racing thoughts. Stressful events are met with feelings of depression or emotional outbursts—road rage, for example. Any of this sound familiar?

The Twenty-First-Century Syndrome: Low Adrenal and Low Thyroid Symptoms

Hypoadrenia, or low adrenal function, is behind many of the problems that we attribute to getting older. Because the adrenal glands produce so many hormones, the symptoms of adrenal fatigue vary, but fatigue that is worse around 3 to 4 p.m. is nearly universally a sign of low adrenal function. You may be thinking, "Hey, isn't everyone tired by then?" No, not if the adrenals are strong. Late-day burnout or depression, particularly during periods of stress—the classic "I just can't cope anymore" feelings—are common symptoms of adrenal depletion. Adrenal symptoms almost always grow worse as the day wears on, or when you feel stressed.

Symptoms of Low Adrenal Function

- Afternoon fatigue and poor endurance
- Irritability, depression (worse with stress)

- Palpitations, anxiety—particularly with stress
- Allergies to food or the environment, or even chemical sensitivity
- Low blood sugar, irritability if meals are delayed, hunger, nausea
- Joint pains; skin irritations (eczema, hives), often in response to stress
- Body aches, headaches, a feeling like a low-grade flu
- Poor concentration, light-headedness
- Headaches, muscle spasm in the upper back/neck/shoulders
- Frequent infections, recurrent yeast infections

Now that you understand a bit about what low adrenal hormones feel like, let's consider thyroid hormones. Every muscle, nerve, and organ in our body requires thyroid hormone to function optimally, so the symptoms of low thyroid hormone are wide-ranging. Thyroid symptoms are typically worse when resting or waking (unlike adrenal symptoms, which usually improve with rest).

People with low thyroid symptoms can look and feel like they've escaped from a twisted fairy tale: grumpy, sleepy, lazy, cold, and over-weight, with a coarse voice and bad hair. (Although many people with low thyroid symptoms can be normal weight or even thin.) They tend to be anxious, and nervous with palpitations and terrible insomnia, due to high noradrenaline. They startle easily and have trouble waking up. In addition, many women with low thyroid have regular menstrual cycles, but the cycles are very heavy, with prolonged bleeding; swollen, tender breasts; and bad PMS due to blunted progesterone (proges-terone receptors that don't work normally when thyroid hormones are low). Bowels are classically constipated, but often there is irregularity with alternating constipation and loose stool. Hair seems to fall off the head, with thinned, shortened eyebrows and thin, listless hair. The mood can be depressed and is often irritable and unpleasant. Low thy-roid hormones cause swelling, especially in the lower legs, with sluggish reflexes. An indented tongue and yellowish palms are also common, and infertility is almost universal.

Signs and Symptoms of Low Thyroid Function

- Fatigue, worse upon rising or resting
- Irritable, depressed mood

- Problems concentrating
- Constipation or erratic bowel movements
- Irregular, heavy, or absent menstrual period
- Weight gain
- Headache, muscle aches
- Poor sleep
- Hair loss or thinning
- Infertility
- Easy bruising
- Puffy eyelids, worse in the morning
- Elevated cholesterol (functional hypothyroid should be ruled out in anyone with elevated cholesterol)
- Elevated blood pressure
- Coarse, dry hair; hair and eyebrow thinning
- Dry, brittle nails; dry skin, "goose flesh" on upper arms
- Swelling of lower legs or hands, yellowed palms or soles
- Cold hands and feet
- Swollen ankles and hands
- Heart disease or heart arrhythmias

How a Normal Thyroid Gland Functions

Your thyroid is controlled by your brain. Your hypothalamus, also known as the "master gland," located in the brain, is governed by your emotions, sexual activity, hunger, thirst, and temperature. It passes this information via the hypothalamic hormone TRH (thyroid-releasing hormone) on to your pituitary gland, located in the very center of your brain (at the end of a very slender stalk, with a blood supply that can be hampered with age and trauma). If you need more thyroid hormone, because you are cold or environmentally stressed, your brain will demand more TSH (thyroid-stimulating hormone) from your pituitary gland, which will then order your thyroid gland to make more thyroid hormone. Once there is enough thyroid hormone, the brain will stop making so much TSH, but if there is not enough thyroid hormone, the TSH level will be high, and if your thyroid gland functions normally, your TSH level will be normal.

Thyroid hormone is made by combining an amino acid (tyrosine) with iodine. The number of iodine molecules will determine what type of thyroid hormone is made and how active the hormone will be. T4 is made of tyrosine with four molecules of iodine, and is largely inactive. It will have little effect on your cells. T3 has three molecules of iodine, and is the active form of thyroid hormone. It is the reason you feel a kick from thyroid hormones.

Most (95 percent) thyroid hormone produced by your thyroid gland is the inactive, T4, form. The activation of T3 from T4 requires the coordinated effort of lots of players. It requires adrenal hormones, particularly DHEA and cortisol; minerals, especially magnesium, selenium, iron, iodine, and copper; and vitamins A, B_2, B_6, B_{12}, and C.

When Thyroid Hormones Aren't Normal

There are many things that can go wrong with your thyroid hormones. The most common problems for women discussed here are problems activating your T4 into T3 (functional low thyroid) or problems with thyroid antibodies.

Functional Low Thyroid

A functional low thyroid means that you feel like your thyroid is low, but everyone who tests you tells you that it's normal. Your gland is working normally, but your cells are not activating your thyroid hormone. If not enough T4 is activated into T3 inside your cells, you will look and feel as though your thyroid production is too low despite routine thyroid blood tests showing normal thyroid hormone (that is, normal T4 and normal TSH). This disorder is very common. People with this problem have all of the signs and symptoms of a low-functioning thyroid gland (fatigue, headache, body aches, heavy menstrual cycles or irregular cycles, dry skin, constipation, moodiness, or depression), but their routine thyroid blood tests are within normal ranges (though usually on the extreme low range of normal; see below).

People with functional low thyroid—and you know who you are—walk around certain that they have a low thyroid condition, but no one believes them. They may be overweight (but can be a normal weight), menstruate too heavily, or have poor circulation or dry, cracking skin. Their bowels are sluggish or erratic, their eyebrows are thinned, and their hair is coarse and dry. They are depressed, achy, and sluggish, and they feel even worse when they rest.

Why does this happen? Well, once again there is likely an evolutionary explanation. Because low thyroid hormones cause serious congenital problems, functional low thyroid may in fact be nature's way of ensuring ideal conditions for pregnancy. The conversion of T4 into T3 requires ideal cell conditions (adequate magnesium, iron, DHEA, cortisol, iodine, and tyrosine). If there is not enough T3, guess what—progesterone, the pregnancy hormone, won't work normally. This is why women with low thyroid hormones have irregular cycles, heavy bleeding, and PMS symptoms. If a woman is low in minerals or food or if her adrenal hormones are low from excess stress or illness, her thyroid will not activate normally. Unless the physical environment is ideal, pregnancy won't take place. Functional low thyroid is nature's very own birth control, which was helpful in the dark ages, but it poses problems for modern-day women.

Most women that I see with heavy menstrual bleeds require thyroid hormone, minerals (particularly iron and magnesium), and vitamin A. Because thyroid hormone is needed to convert beta-carotene into vitamin A, you must use a vitamin A form of replacement (not one made from beta-carotene). High doses of vitamin A are often needed to treat bleeding problems, as vitamin A strengthens the uterine lining. (I usually recommend 50,000 U per day, which is safe for three to six months if you have normal liver function.) High doses should be taken only with a doctor's guidance and typically for only two to three months. More and more infertility doctors are recognizing the interaction between thyroid hormone and progesterone, and many clinics now require women going through infertility treatments to maintain their TSH between 1 and 2.

Causes of Functional Low Thyroid

1. **Magnesium deficiency**   Magnesium is the most common mineral deficiency, and is a frequent cause of low thyroid function. I would estimate that nearly 40 percent of my new patients are mildly or severely magnesium-deficient. Symptoms of low magnesium are: headache, intolerance to bright light, irritability, fatigue, and menstrual cramps.

2. **Iron deficiency**   Iron deficiency is common in women with heavy bleeds. I always try to have low thyroid patients maintain their ferritin above 60 ng/ml.

3. **Low adrenal hormones**, particularly DHEA and cortisol (discussed later).

4. **Medications that can interfere with T4 activation**   NSAIDs (nonsteroidal anti-inflammatory drugs such as Ibuprofen and Naprosyn), birth control pills, oral estrogen, chemotherapy (interferon, 5FU, tamoxifen, 6-mercaptopurine), most antidepressants and sleeping pills, beta-blockers, lithium, phenytoin, amiodarone, and theophylline.

5. **Toxins**, including pesticides, mercury, fluoride, radiation, alcohol, caffeine, cigarette smoke, and phthalates (chemicals added to plastics, often emitted when heating or microwaving plastics).

6. **Thyroid antibodies**   These are discussed below.

Thyroid Antibodies

Thyroid antibodies are also a common problem for perimenopausal and menopausal women, and you should know if you have any. Autoimmune thyroiditis, also known as Hashimoto's disease, is fifty times more common in women than in men, and tends to occur during perimenopause and menopause. Auto-antibodies are proteins made by your white blood cells that damage other parts of your body. Thyroid antibodies can do many things to your thyroid gland or thyroid hormones: (1) Inflame your gland so that excess hormones are made. (2) Damage your thyroid gland so that not enough thyroid hormones are made. (3) Interfere with your thyroid receptors so your hormones don't act normally. (4) Interfere with T4 activation.

Antibodies are common, and you can determine if you have them by checking a blood test. Do this especially if your TSH is greater than 2.0 mU/ml. It is not clear why antibodies form. Some researchers believe that infections may be a cause; others blame diet or food allergies, particularly to foods containing gluten. Gluten is a protein found in wheat, rye, barley, and oats. It is estimated that 3 to 5 percent of people with autoimmune thyroid disease may be gluten-sensitive, and their symptoms improve on a gluten-free diet.

Thyroid antibodies increase and decrease over time and don't always cause low-thyroid complaints. In fact, sometimes your thyroid gland can become overstimulated (hyperthyroid) from auto-antibodies, and other times your gland can appear perfectly normal. The presence of thyroid antibodies can help predict how long you will need thyroid hormone support. In my experience, people who don't have thyroid antibodies and need some thyroid support usually don't need it for long. Their thyroid is not functioning well because of a deficiency of a particular nutrient, and replacing the deficient mineral, hormone, or vitamins will suffice.

Bread, Salt, and Iodine Deficiency

Iodine deficiency is the most common cause of thyroid problems worldwide, and there is growing concern about iodine deficiency in the United States. It all has to do with bread and salt.

Iodine is a major component of thyroid hormones. We need at least 150 mcg per day (200 to 250 mcg/day if pregnant or breast-feeding). Iodine deficiency, in addition to making us grow cranky and cold with goiters (enlarged thyroid glands), lowers thyroid hormone levels. If that happens during pregnancy, babies are born not as smart as they could be (the medical term for this is "cretinism"). In the 1920s, to avoid this problem, iodine was added to our salt and our bread (after it was noted that 40 percent of people living in Michigan, where the soil was iodine-deficient, were found to have developed goiters). Before 1960, each slice of bread contained 150 mcg of iodine, and the average American consumed 1 mg of iodine daily (75 percent of this from baked products).

In the 1960s, fears that this was excessive led to the substitution of bromide for iodide. This loss of bread iodide (a form of iodine), coupled with an increase in bromide and trends toward low-salt/no-salt diets and natural unfortified salts, has brought about a new problem, breast disease.

Both our mammary glands (breasts) and our thyroid glands have been linked from the time we were embryos and both have a special ability to store iodine. This function is vital during pregnancy and breast-feeding. Because bromide has been replacing iodide in our bread and in our breasts for the past fifty years, it is feared that this has led to an increase in both breast cancer and fibrocystic breast disease (both of which have increased dramatically over this time period).

There are several supports for this theory: (1) The Japanese have the highest iodine content in their diet and the lowest rates of breast cancer and breast disease. The Japanese consume nearly 12 mg of iodine daily, mostly from seafood and seaweeds (like those used in sushi, for example), as compared with North Americans, who consume 150 to 200 mcg per day or less. (2) Fibrocystic breast disease improves with iodine therapy (see below). (3) Iodine protects breast cells from precancerous states (dysplasia) and carcinogens. (4) Iodine is an antioxidant, and antioxidants are known to lower the risk of breast cancer. (5) Women with goiters have an increased risk of breast cancer. (6) Iodine deficiency is associated with an increased risk of breast cancer. There is a theory that lack of iodine causes the breast cells to become more sensitive to estrogen stimulation. Studies have shown that both thyroid supplementation and iodine use reduce fibrocystic changes in the breast and reduce cysts in the ovaries.

Iodine can be measured with a twenty-four-hour urine test. A quick, simple test that I like to do with my patients is to paint a patch of tincture of iodine (available at most drugstores) on their inner upper arm and see how long it takes for the resulting brown circle to disappear. If it is gone within two hours, I assume that the patient is very deficient. If she has enough iodine, her patch will still be seen on her arm after twenty-four hours. The longer it takes to disappear, the better her stores. If your skin patch is gone before twenty-four hours, I recommend supplementing with iodine and increasing iodine-rich foods in your diet. Seafood is a great source of iodine. All seaweeds are high in iodine (brown and red are highest), and you will get iodine from eating many types of sushi. I also recommend using kelp as a seasoning. Fish from the sea (particularly sea bass and cod) are better sources than freshwater fish.

Iodine is tricky. You need enough to make thyroid hormone, but if you take too much, you could reduce your ability to release thyroid hormone from your gland. Years ago, iodine was the standard treatment for an overactive thyroid. For these reasons, iodine supplementation is considered somewhat controversial. But as with all things, taken in moderation, iodine is safe and effective, particularly if you suffer from fibrocystic breast disease or have problems making enough thyroid hormone. The usual dose that I recommend for fibrocystic breast problems is 1 to 3 mg daily (some women who are very deficient may need more, 4 to 5 mg/day). Naturally, I would advise using high doses only with your doctor's guidance, and you should monitor you thyroid function while doing so. Elemental iodine has been shown to be better than using iodide. If you simply want to supplement iodine, use 150 to 200 mcg daily.

Measuring Your Thyroid Hormones

Now that you have a basic understanding of how your thyroid gland functions normally, and what can go wrong, you need to be familiar with some tests that can help determine if you have a thyroid problem. Most routine tests do not measure free thyroid hormones or T3 levels. Here is a list of thyroid tests that you can request:

> **TSH blood test**   This is the most common test most doctors use to detect low thyroid function. When your thyroid is functioning normally, your TSH will not be high. But if your thyroid hormones are too low, your TSH rises, attempting to produce more thyroid hormones. So an elevated TSH level is a sure sign that thyroid hormone levels are low. This is counterintuitive: if the test result is high, you need more hormone, not less. The higher the TSH level, the lower the thyroid hormone level, and vice versa.
>
> In many circumstances TSH tests will be unreliable. Aging, sleep deprivation, excess stress, depression, anxiety, low-calorie diets, cancer, diabetes, kidney disease, or overuse of alcohol can all affect TSH function. Medications such as lipid-lowering drugs, oral contraceptives, antidepressants, contrast agents (dyes used in some X rays), and antihistamines can also affect TSH testing. Whenever TSH production is not functioning properly, the TSH level will be normal or may even be low, despite low thyroid hormone production or low thyroid activation inside your cells. If this is happening, the diagnosis of low thyroid will be missed. To complicate matters further, TSH tests can sometimes be misinterpreted. Here are two problems interpreting TSH:
>
> 1. **The true healthy range for TSH is in dispute.** There is debate among doctors and in medical journals about the cor-

rect normal ranges for TSH. In fact, some doctors choose to ignore the TSH level. Laboratories vary, but most labs report the normal range for TSH as between 0.5 and 5.5 mU/l. This is a very broad range. Many doctors feel that TSH is best between 1 and 2 mU/l, and I use this as the normal range for my patients. If your TSH is over 2.0 mU/l, this is usually a sign that there is a problem with thyroid hormone production or activation, and thyroid support will help your symptoms. Once treated, monitor your TSH. When your thyroid is corrected, your TSH will begin to fall. I maintain my patients' TSH between 1 and 2. Once TSH falls below 1.0 mU/l, you can usually start to withdraw thyroid support slowly.

2. **TSH is not always reliable.** If your TSH is normal and you nevertheless have many signs or symptoms of low thyroid function, take a twenty-four-hour urine thyroid test to measure how much thyroid is inside your cells in a twenty-four-hour period. This test will often show low levels of active T3 that were not detected by the indirect TSH blood measurements. Always remember that how you feel is more important than any test result.

Free T4 and free T3 tests   T3 levels are often ignored by many doctors, but your T3 level is important. Both T4 and T3 can be measured from your blood, or from a twenty-four-hour urine test. (See chapter 6 for the names of laboratories that provide these.) I use both, but blood level results have limited value, as they are only a snapshot in time. Because your thyroid is most active during the day, a daytime blood draw may test high but your thyroid function may be too low when you are not active. If your T3 is very low but your T4 is normal, you likely have a problem converting T4 into T3, and treatment with T3 and/or herbs and minerals to improve T4 activation will be helpful.

Twenty-four-hour urine tests   These tests avoid daytime variations in hormone levels and should be done if you have many signs and symptoms of low thyroid but your TSH and free levels of thyroid hormones are normal. I have found them particularly useful for people who look and feel as if their thyroid is too low but whose blood tests are normal.

Other Tests

Iron levels, or ferritin　There are various forms of iron; serum iron differs from stored iron. It is the stored form, or ferritin, that most affects thyroid conversion. You want your ferritin level over 60 ng/ml (10 to 330 ng/ml) for optimal thyroid function.

RBC magnesium　Magnesium is the most common mineral deficiency seen in adults. Magnesium deficiency may be caused by chronic stress, poor diet, or chronic yeast infections. Magnesium is found inside our blood cells and is needed to activate T4 thyroid hormone into T3. To properly test magnesium, you must check the level of magnesium inside the cells. Do this by measuring an RBC (red blood cell) magnesium level. The level should be midrange or above. A simple blood serum test for magnesium will not do, because magnesium is primarily found inside the cells and not in the serum. Checking only the serum level will miss most deficiencies.

DHEA-S and cortisol　Both of these adrenal hormones can be measured from the blood, urine, or saliva and should be midrange or above—if DHEA is too low or cortisol levels are too high, thyroid hormones and thyroid activation can be suppressed.

Thyroid antibodies　Thyroid antibodies are not normally present, and it is significant when they are detected. Their presence usually indicates that thyroid hormones will be needed long-term. If you test positive, but your thyroid function is normal, I would retest thyroid hormone levels each year, and more frequently if symptoms change.

How Normal Adrenal Glands Function

Although there are over forty adrenal hormones, there are only a few that you really need to care about: cortisol, aldosterone, DHEA, adrenaline (epinephrine), and pregnenolone.

When you are under stress, the pituitary gland in your brain releases ACTH (adrenocorticotropic hormone), which triggers your adrenal glands to get working. Each adrenal gland promptly produces adrenaline (epinephrine) from the inside (the medulla) of the gland and pregnenolone, DHEA, cortisol, and aldosterone from its outer side (the cortex).

All hormones from the adrenal gland's cortex are made from cholesterol. From cholesterol comes a cascade of hormones, as shown in the diagram below. The Chinese liken our liver metabolism of these adrenal hormones to a flowing stream. The stream can be gently moving, or flooding if there are "rocks" and "boulders" in its path. Many toxins, such as alcohol and caffeine and even medications, can disrupt this natural flow of hormones. I see this all of the time when I am interpreting hormone metabolites with my

Adrenal Hormone Cascade

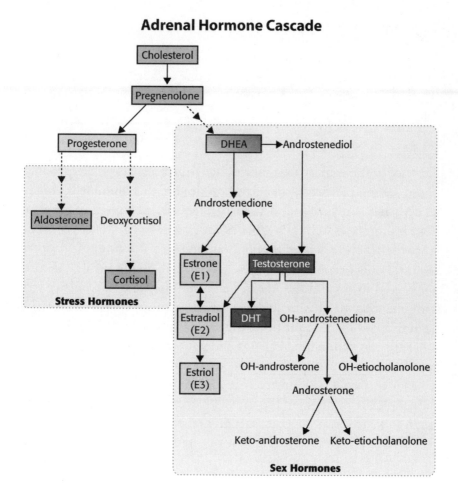

patients. For instance, if I give a woman DHEA, it should ideally flow "downward" in a cascade (much like the Chinese describe, as "flowing streams" in the liver) into various metabolites, eventually forming testosterone or estrogen. When I interpret hormone metabolites, if I see a combination of some very high metabolite levels with some very low metabolite levels, I know that liver metabolism is uneven, out of balance—what Chinese medicine describes as "stuck liver qi." It is as if there were rocks and downed trees blocking the liver flow of hormones. So I prescribe liver herbs to help the hormones flow better. This image also explains why sometimes women have high DHEA levels, even though they are not using any supplemental DHEA. Their DHEA is "stuck," not being metabolized. Often this causes complaints such as headache and irritability.

Your Adrenal Hormones

Our adrenal hormones support our energy, endurance, and immune function. Signs and symptoms of hormone deficiencies or excesses are listed in appendixes A and B. Here's what you need to know about the major adrenal hormones.

Cortisol

Cortisol is the major stress hormone. Your body normally produces about 20 mg of cortisol per day, and double this amount if you are under stress. Cortisol supports energy, reduces inflammation, controls your immune system, and regulates your sugar levels. Many people are warned that cortisol is an immune suppressant. But immune suppression will only occur at high doses, greater than 20 mg per day. If cortisol is used in small doses, it can be taken safely and will bolster your immune system. This is unlike synthetic cortisol substitutes such as prednisone, which is four times more potent than cortisol. Prednisone will suppress your adrenal glands and your immune function. For this reason it is used to stop allergic or severe autoimmune reactions.

Your cortisol level is normally highest first thing in the morning and falls gradually throughout the day (with occasional small jumps around noon and 3 to 4 p.m.). As cortisol falls as the day goes on, you eventually feel tired by nighttime. This is how our natural circadian rhythm normally works: high cortisol in the morning and low cortisol at night, ris-

Cortisol Curves

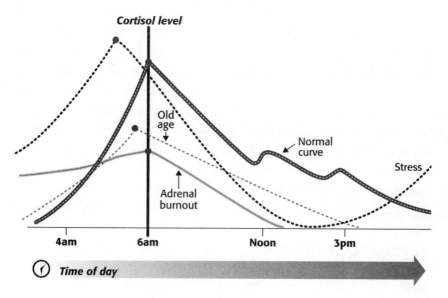

ing again at the time of waking the next day. With chronic stress, adrenal deficiency, shift work, chronic insomnia, overwork, and age, you can lose your cortisol control and have low morning levels and high evening or nighttime levels, causing overeating, weight gain, and insomnia.

Cortisol curves can be measured by testing saliva levels throughout the day and night. This can be helpful in figuring out why you are tired or restless at a certain time of day, or why you can't sleep at night. If your morning cortisol is low, then by 2 or 3 p.m. there may be little if any cortisol left to fuel your afternoon, causing a "slump" at 3 or 4 p.m. You may see an afternoon and evening rise, turning you into a night owl. Night owls often report afternoon fatigue with a second wind late in the day, and then a hard time winding down for bed.

As we age, our morning cortisol production is lower and starts earlier, around 5 a.m. This partly explains why older people tend to wake earlier and run out of steam more easily. If cortisol control is poor, with rises too early or too late, I usually recommend using a supplement known as phosphatidylserine or phosphoserine (100 to 300 mg throughout the day or at bedtime).

To help you understand, look at the cortisol curves shown above.

DHEA

DHEA is the most abundant hormone in your body. It is important for stabilizing mood, helping to activate thyroid hormone, building bone, deepening sleep, and improving memory and sex drive. It was once thought that it was an intermediary hormone whose sole task was to make other hormones, and that it had no function of its own, but we now know otherwise. Think of DHEA as a battery providing the body with energy and stamina. DHEA stimulates the production of serotonin, cortisol, and sex hormones, particularly estrogen and testosterone, in women. It is used to treat osteoporosis, depression, obesity, heart disease, sexual dysfunction, dementia, and autoimmune disease. Men do not form testosterone from DHEA, but women do, and I prescribe DHEA right away to women with a low sex drive and low testosterone levels. It is less expensive and has fewer side effects than testosterone.

People with low DHEA complain that they no longer dream or sleep deeply or that they have a great tendency to catch colds and the flu. They tend to have aches and pains and are prone to bone loss. Weight gain is common with low DHEA, with a tendency to develop a flabby belly and cellulite. Because women make testosterone (and estrogen) from DHEA, it is vital for a healthy sex drive. If your DHEA level is low, you may notice that your pubic hair and underarm hair are scant and your skin has a tendency to be very dry, appearing somewhat pale and lusterless. A unique but consistent symptom of low DHEA is intolerance to loud noises.

Pregnenolone

Pregnenolone is the mother of all hormones because it produces sex hormones and stress hormones (as shown in the adrenal cascade). It is the major adrenal hormone of the brain, where its levels are thirty times higher than in the blood. It plays an important role in helping to balance your neurotransmitters and improve your memory. Symptoms of low pregnenolone are varied and look like low adrenal function (fatigue, low blood pressure, poor resistance to stress or infection, and poor memory). Some people describe feeling like their brain is too slow, not as quick or sharp as it used to be. They may notice a lower sex drive or PMS symptoms because pregnenolone produces sex hormones, progesterone in particular.

Aldosterone

Aldosterone helps to control blood pressure. It maintains blood flow to our brain so that we can think on our feet during emergencies. People with low aldosterone complain of dizzy spells when they get up quickly and drowsiness if they have to sit upright or stand too long. You can spot a person with low aldosterone—they are the ones falling asleep at the exciting movies. When your aldosterone is low, you usually feel best lying flat, and you may find yourself announcing when you come home after a long day, "I just need to put my feet up."

When aldosterone is low, blood pressure readings are often too low and can fall below 100 (the systolic, or top number). Often such people are told that they have a great blood pressure because it is so low. But as with all things, too high or too low is not good, particularly a low blood pressure accompanied by dizziness. Other symptoms of low aldosterone are thirst, frequent urination, or the feeling that whatever you drink goes right through you. If your aldosterone is low, you are easily dehydrated.

If your aldosterone is too high, your blood pressure will be elevated, which is common with chronic stress and is one reason that stress is related to hypertension. When you are chronically stressed, your brain is constantly pumping out ACTH to stimulate your adrenal glands to make stress hormones, particularly adrenaline and cortisol. Over time only that part of the adrenal gland that makes aldosterone responds to the ACTH. So your aldosterone may rise, but cortisol and adrenaline may actually fall. Unfortunately, people are often put on medications to lower their aldosterone (which does lower the blood pressure), but really what they need is to strengthen their adrenal glands. Once cortisol is restored, stress is better handled, aldosterone usually returns to normal, and blood pressure readings fall. If you have high blood pressure, ask your doctor to check your aldosterone (before starting medications that will blunt your results). Taking diuretics or blood pressure medications may not treat the root of your problem; weakened adrenals and overcompensating high aldosterone may go untreated.

Epinephrine

Epinephrine (EPI), which is the same as adrenaline, is made by the medulla, the innermost part of the adrenal gland. Epinephrine is our "first responder" hormone to stress. It is vital to be able to cope with sudden and immediate stress. I would routinely use it in the ER to revive a patient whose heart has stopped beating. It is a life-or-death hormone, but it also flows in our bloodstream every minute of every day, giving us energy and stamina and balancing our emotions. Like thyroid hormone, it is made from tyrosine; and it is balanced by another neurotransmitter, norepinephrine (NE), which actually makes EPI. Estrogen derives much of its kick by helping to maintain EPI and NE levels (progesterone lowers both of these). Low EPI and low NE levels are implicated in depression, and contribute to the mood swings seen when estradiol levels begin to fall during perimenopause.

Measuring Adrenal Hormones

You can measure your adrenal hormones (and hormone metabolites) with blood, urine, or saliva tests. To determine how well the adrenal gland is functioning, I typically measure and monitor the adrenal hormones discussed above: cortisol, pregnenolone, DHEA, aldosterone, and adrenaline (epinephrine).

Cortisol

- **Cortisol blood tests** are tricky to interpret since cortisol varies with the time of day and stress levels. For this reason a blood cortisol level has limited value (but if you do measure it, do so first thing in the morning, when it is peaking. This level should be between 15 and 22 ug/dl). Late-afternoon or evening levels should be on the lowest end of the normal range to enable a person to wind down and fall asleep, usually 3 to 7ug/dl.
- **Salivary cortisol** can be measured throughout the day to see how well your cortisol is regulated. Remember, you want your cortisol to be highest in the morning, with a gradual decline as the day goes on.
- **A twenty-four-hour urine test for cortisol** can be helpful to determine how severe your cortisol deficiency might be. I prefer this test to a morning cortisol measurement because it takes into account the ups and downs of cortisol production and gives you a twenty-four-hour average. If your twenty-four-hour urine cor-

tisol is less than 50 ug per twenty-four hours, I recommend using a strong support such as bioidentical cortisol itself. If your level is over 50 ug per twenty-four hours, I recommend a milder support (adrenal extract or herbal support)—but more on this later. If you are taking a twenty-four-hour urine test for cortisol, it is important to avoid any stress or exertion that will raise your cortisol levels; otherwise you will miss detecting a cortisol deficiency.

- **A cortisol stimulation test** is considered the gold standard for diagnosing adrenal insufficiency. This test involves giving an injection of ACTH (pituitary hormone that stimulates the adrenal glands) and measuring how much cortisol is made. Your cortisol level should double in response to the ACTH. This test was developed to detect the very rare condition Addison's disease, an advanced state of adrenal depletion in which 90 percent of the adrenal glands are destroyed or not functioning. This test will not detect the common, less severe adrenal deficiency, hypoadrenia. Such people test normally on a stimulation test, but they are walking around with very low daytime cortisol levels (and/or high evening cortisol) and feel chronically tired, anxious, and depressed. They do not have Addison's disease, but they chronically underproduce cortisol and often fail to regulate their cortisol normally.

Pregnenolone

Pregnenolone blood tests can be helpful but it is hard to know what the best level is, since pregnenolone is constantly changing, converting into other adrenal hormones as needed. I measure this to determine if adrenal reserves are very low. Look for a morning blood pregnenolone level to be over 30 ng/dl (10 to 230 ng/dl). It is important to avoid stress and excess exertion in the twenty-four-hour period prior to the blood draw, because it will be higher than normal.

DHEA

- **The blood DHEA-sulfate (DHEA-S) level** should be measured because this is the most abundant and most stable form of DHEA circulating. I look at this level as your reserves, and seek to maintain it in the upper midrange of normal. The level should not be too high or too low. If you are told that your level is fine but you don't feel fine, look closely at the actual value. You may see that your level is well below midrange. This implies a low DHEA reserve and indicates a need for DHEA replacement, particularly if you have symptoms of low DHEA, low testosterone, or bone loss. I recommend that my menopausal patients maintain their DHEA-S at around 120 to 150 pg/ml, even though the normal range for a fifty-year-old woman is 15 to 170 pg/ml. As you age, it will normally fall, but the goal is to maintain hormone balance, and DHEA will sustain all of your bones and your sex hormones as you grow older, so keep it midrange, or slightly above.

- **Twenty-four-hour urine tests for DHEA and its metabolites** are a great way to follow DHEA therapy to ensure that DHEA is acting safely inside your body. DHEA breaks down in your liver into many metabolites. If your liver is busy breaking down drugs, alcohol, or caffeine, it may not convert DHEA well. When this happens, DHEA and DHEA metabolite levels can rise. In the short term this can result in headaches and irritability. The long-term effects are not well understood, but could pose additional problems. Remember, the goal is always to restore levels to normal, not excessive, and to avoid excessive metabolite levels.
- **Saliva tests for DHEA** can be helpful and less expensive, particularly if you are measuring saliva for other hormones.

Aldosterone

Blood or twenty-four-hour aldosterone levels may be measured. The level of aldosterone is naturally higher when in the upright position for a prolonged period of time. For this reason, twenty-four-hour levels may be a more accurate measure, but I see plenty of abnormal first-morning blood levels.

Epinephrine

Urine tests for epinephrine are typically done two hours after waking, when epinephrine levels are peaking. I also check epinephrine levels in a night urine test if there is trouble falling asleep or waking during the night.

Supporting Low Thyroid or Adrenal Hormones

There are many ways to treat adrenal and thyroid hormones using herbs, hormones, extracts, vitamins, and minerals. Treat if you have symptoms of deficiency and treat whatever hormones are low or below the midrange of normal. Don't wait for hormone deficiency to weaken your body further. I usually support adrenal hormones first, wait a few days to see what effect that has, and then add any thyroid support needed. Using multiple adrenal hormones and/or herbs in low doses usually works well and avoids the unwanted side effects of high doses. For example, if DHEA, pregnenolone, and cortisol are low or below midrange, support them all in as low a dose as possible to feel the most balanced. How you feel will be the true test. Expect to feel as good as you used to feel when you were younger. Whatever you start with, wait a couple of days to see what symptoms improve. Both adrenal and thyroid hormones are stimulating, but should improve your sleep. If sleep is disturbed, it is a sign that you need to decrease something. Don't change more than one thing at a time, or it will be difficult to tell what's working and what's not.

Strengthening Your Adrenals

Deciding the best way to strengthen and support your adrenal glands depends on how your adrenals are doing, how you are feeling, and how you react to medications and supplements in general. Some people are very sensitive, and for them a little goes a long way. Start with a very low dose of whatever support you are going to use and increase it as needed until you start to feel better. Almost immediately you should notice that your energy is improved and more consistent, without dips in the day. As your energy becomes more stable, your mood will also stabilize, and your tired, irritable feelings will leave. You will have more patience because you're not feeling so wiped out.

There are many ways to treat adrenal fatigue, and I like to think of adrenal supports in tiers, like a wedding cake. The strongest, most potent support is cortisol; next are adrenal extracts; below that are stimulating herbs such as ginseng, and then less energizing herbs such as rhodiola, ginkgo, and licorice root. Least noticeable but also effective are vitamin supports such as vitamin C, pantothenic acid, PABA (para-aminobenzoic acid), and other B vitamins. Tyrosine and SAMe can be used to support epinephrine in particular.

Using Bioidentical Cortisol

Of all the hormones that I recommend to improve quality of life, bioidentical cortisol is probably the most controversial. This is because cortisol has taken on a scary, dangerous aura. Yes, it is potent and must be used with care, but it is not the same as other very potent synthetic forms of cortisol (prednisone and prednisilone), which have been overused and are four times stronger than bioidentical cortisol. These steroids lower DHEA levels and are often prescribed in very high dosages (to suppress the body's response to inflammation). This leads to frequent side effects such as high blood pressure, a weakened immune system, weight gain, bloating, diabetes, stomach ulcers, bone loss, and even mania.

Bioidentical cortisol (Cortef, or hydrocortisone) is natural; that is, it is chemically, structurally, and in every way the same as the hydocortisone normally produced by your adrenal glands every day. Used in small, physiologic doses, natural cortisol will support and strengthen your adrenals. Cortisol dramatically improves fatigue, depression, body aches, and repeated infections. It is not for everyone, but if you have very low adrenal function and significant symptoms, it can turn your life around. I recommend it for people with severe fatigue or depression symptoms whose morning blood level of cortisol is less than 10 ug/dl or whose twenty-four-hour urine cortisol level is less than 50 ug in twenty-four hours.

One of the best features of cortisol is that its effects are immediate. Within hours you should notice more energy, improved mood, and a greater sense of well-being. Cortisol should be taken at the same time of day that it is normally produced by your body, first thing in the morning. You may need another dose at noon, and possibly a third dose in the later afternoon, between 3 and 4 p.m. A late dose is especially helpful if your day is expected to be particularly stressful or long. Never take cortisol later than 3 or 4 p.m., since this is not when your body would naturally produce it and taking it this late will interfere with your sleep.

Cortisol dosing is very individualized and can even change from day to day. Most people find that 5 to 15 mg per day of cortisol is usually all that is needed. At these small doses, the adrenals will not be suppressed or weakened. Remember, your goal is to take only what your body should be making, not an excess amount. Your body normally produces 15 to 20 mg per day, and 20 to 40 mg per day when stressed or ill. Always start with as low a dose as needed and increase the dose slowly. I usually start most patients with 2.5 to 5 mg in the morning and 2.5 to 5 mg at noon, and see how they feel. If they are still fatigued, I will then increase the dose by 2.5 to 5 mg. If you feel anxious or hyper on your dose, reduce it the next day by 2.5 to 5 mg.

You need to play with the dose, but with time you will know what you need. Cortisol acts quickly, and your dose should be adjusted downward if you feel overly energetic or if you start to have any insomnia. Conversely, if you feel sluggish, your dose should be increased (usually by 2.5 or 5 mg). If you are sick or stressed, you should increase your dose. I usually have patients double their morning dose and increase their afternoon dose by half if they are regularly using cortisol and become sick or suffer extreme stress. It is fine to change the dose as needed, so long as you don't use doses greater than 15 to 20 mg per day on a regular basis. Doses consistently above 20 mg a day will suppress or weaken your adrenal glands and cause you to be more susceptible to illness or stress.

Cortisol is not intended to be used forever. Usually after two to four months, most people notice their cortisol is making them too energetic or anxious, or they are having trouble sleeping. These are signs that they need less. Whether and when you will be ready to cut back depends on many things, such as how low your adrenal function was to begin with, and how much stress (illness or emotional/physical stress) persists in your life. If you are uncertain, a repeat of your twenty-four-hour urine test or a cortisol blood test may help decide whether to reduce your support. Always lower your dose gradually, and when you do cut back, you will need to use a less strong adrenal support (discussed below). I usually lower the afternoon dose first. If you feel fatigued or depressed on a lower dose, don't reduce it. Maintain your cortisol level, but figure out why you have persistent adrenal fatigue. Common causes are life stress (overwork, excessive travel, inadequate rest or vacation, emotional turmoil), persistent infections (chronic yeast, parasites, Lyme disease, chronic viral infections), recurrent illnesses, heavy metal poisoning, or toxic exposures.

Side effects should not occur if cortisol is used properly. Always take cortisol with food and don't use it in excessive doses. Cortisol stimulates stomach acid, which is one reason that people under stress may develop stomach ulcers. Cortisol should not be used with anti-inflammatory medications.

Common side effects of taking too much cortisol are anxiety, palpitations, and difficulty sleeping. Cortisol can stimulate your appetite, so be careful not to gain weight on it. This shouldn't happen if you are using the right dose. Cortisol can cause swelling of your ankles and/or a rise in blood pressure, and too much cortisol will lower your thyroid function. Bone loss is a frequent problem with synthetic cortisol (prednisone) but should not occur in low-dose, short-term therapies of cortisol.

One of cortisol's roles is to help your body retain sodium and lose potassium to help maintain blood pressure in times of emergency. So blood pressure should improve—that is, become higher if too low and become lower if too high. Naturally, your doctor should guide your treatment and monitor your blood pressure and body salts. When using cortisol, if any swelling occurs, potassium aspartate (100 to 400 mg/day) should be taken, and swelling will usually lessen.

Cortisol normally functions to raise blood sugar and blood pressure needed by your body to cope with emergencies. This should not be a problem with doses below 15 mg a day. You should be sure to monitor your blood pressure and your sugar if you have a diabetic tendency.

Using DHEA

Your optimal **DHEA** dose depends on how low your level is, what your symptoms are, and how well your liver metabolizes it. Most women need only small doses (2 to 15 mg/day) but sometimes, if you are very deficient, you may need as much as 25 or even 50 mg/day. These high doses are typically what you will find in most health food stores, so be aware when shopping what dose you are buying.

DHEA is generally taken in the morning, particularly if you have symptoms of low energy. If you have trouble sleeping as well, you should begin to notice that your sleep is deepening after a couple of weeks, as your DHEA levels are restoring. Occasionally I will recommend a small nighttime dose (not more than 5 to 10 mg) at bedtime to further improve sleep. Sometimes a nighttime dose can disturb your sleep, and if this happens, simply take your entire dose in the morning.

Usually after a period of a few months your DHEA can be reduced, but do this gradually. If, when reducing your DHEA, you notice that your sleep is not as deep, your mood is not as good, your sex drive is not as strong, or your energy or stamina is not what it was, don't reduce your dose but do try to figure out why you still need DHEA support. Most people who become DHEA-deficient are just too busy. If your levels are persistently low, look at your lifestyle. Where is the stress? How much sleep and rest are you allowing yourself? Are you working too hard? Are you taking regular vacations? Drinking too much caffeine? Getting enough or too much exercise? High-performance athletes and marathoners are prone to low DHEA levels, as are busy executives and overworked moms.

Because DHEA can convert into other hormones, you need to keep an eye on your metabolites via twenty-four-hour urine tests. Your doctor can help you to understand how DHEA is working in you. Possible side effects of DHEA are greasy skin, acne, oily hair, an increase in facial or body hair, hair loss, or excess body odor. These side effects are caused from DHEA converting into androstanedione and are usually not seen until after many months of use. Just as testosterone can make too much DHT from the enzyme reductase, this same enzyme can convert DHEA into androstandedione. How active your reductase enzyme is is largely determined by your genetics. Typically women who are naturally prone to excess facial and body hair have more reductase activity and are more prone to making this bothersome metabolite.

Your DHEA and your androstanedione levels can be measured from your blood or urine. Excess androstanedione usually happens from too high a dose of DHEA, poor liver metabolism of DHEA at any dose, or luck of the draw in the gene lottery. If you are concerned about hair loss with DHEA use, be sure to measure these levels before and during treatment to see if it is being affected. You may want to use a ketosteroid form of DHEA (dehydrone form, available as either a 5 mg, 15 mg, or 25 mg dose), as it is less likely to metabolize into androstanedione. If your androstanedione level rises, lower your DHEA or take a break from using it. Zinc (50 to 60 mg/day), saw palmetto (160 to 320 mg/day), and progesterone (200 mg/day, cycled with your cycle) all help to limit androstanedione levels by reducing reductase activity. Avoiding or limiting foods and drugs that are a burden on the liver will also help. This means reducing your intake of alcohol, caffeine, hormones taken by mouth, and most prescription medications. Exercise also helps, particularly brisk aerobic activities. Lower your DHEA dose, say to 2 to 5 mg per day, and pulse it in. That is, use it for two to three months, give yourself a break for a month or two, and reintroduce it as needed and as your body tolerates it without side effects.

Reducing the dose will fix any unwanted side effects such as insomnia, excessive (nervous) energy, or palpitations. Some people are very sensitive to DHEA, and if palpitations or excitability occurs, your pharmacist can compound a slow-release form of DHEA.

Using Pregnenolone

Pregnenolone is available over the counter in the United States, but, like DHEA, it is usually sold in doses that are too high and in forms that are poorly or erratically absorbed. I usually prescribe pregnenolone in low doses, usually 5 to 10 mg per day. Because pregnenolone is so high up in the hormone production chain, it can convert into cortisol, progesterone, DHEA, testosterone, and estrogen. One benefit of pregnenolone over DHEA is that it is less likely to cause acne, facial hair, or hair thinning.

Pregnenolone doses of 5 to 10 mg per day are usually sufficient in both men and women, but if your level is very low or you have a lot of fatigue symptoms, use 20 to 30 mg per day. Always take it in the morning because it is so energizing. It is best absorbed on an empty stomach.

Side effects of pregnenolone are dose-related. If your dose is too high, your sleep will be disturbed or you will feel anxious or hyper, or have palpitations. Pregnenolone is safe as long as your dose is not too high. Animal studies with high doses have failed to show any major side effects. Because it is can convert into other adrenal and sex hormones, it may be necessary to use lower doses of DHEA and cortisol when using it.

Supporting Aldosterone

Aldosterone quickly regulates blood pressure and blood flow to our brain when we are stressed or on our feet too long. As hormones go, its effects are very short-lived, lasting about twenty minutes. Not even the most dedicated hormone enthusiast would be willing to dose this frequently. For this reason, although bioidentical aldosterone is available from some compounding pharmacies, this is one time I would consider using its synthetic sister, Florinef, or the less potent, natural knockoff, licorice root. Both improve the symptoms of low aldosterone. Both raise cortisol, which behaves like aldosterone and lowers aldosterone levels. Both raise blood pressure and lower potassium.

Florinef effects last all day, and it is generally well tolerated and safely metabolized. It can improve endurance and energy in chronic fatigue patients, particularly if they have very low blood pressure (below 100 systolic). Florinef is available by prescription in tablets of 0.1 mg. A typical dose is one half to one tablet (0.05 to 0.1 mg) daily. When using it, you should notice better stamina and more consistent energy. It should not be taken if you have a history of high blood pressure, and it should be used cautiously if you are prone to ankle swelling or fluid retention in general (see below).

Licorice root has been used for centuries by many cultures for adrenal fatigue. It contains an active ingredient known as glycyrrhenic acid, which blocks the breakdown of cortisol into cortisone and makes cortisol more active at aldosterone receptors, acting like aldosterone. The dose varies, depending on the glycrrhenic acid content. Typical daily doses are 250 to 900 mg of dry powdered extract, 2 to 4 ml of a liquid extract, or 1 to 2 gm of powdered root. It is usually taken in two to three doses throughout the day.

The side effects of licorice and Florinef are high blood pressure, low potassium, and swelling. These effects are due to excess cortisol. Monitor your blood pressure, sodium, and potassium every three to six months. If swelling or high blood pressure occurs, notify your doctor, lower or stop the treatment, and take potassium. I often recommend taking 100 to 200 mg of potassium aspartate daily to avoid fluid retention when using adrenal supplements. Most fruits and vegetables are high in potassium, so eating a healthy diet is also important.

Supporting Epinephrine

Epinephrine is the most potent of all adrenal supports, and is used in hospital emergency departments routinely for treating cardiac arrest and severe allergic reactions. Because it is so strong and short-lived, it is never used for symptoms of mere fatigue. Epinephrine can be supported by using the amino acid tyrosine. Tyrosine supports both excitatory neurotransmitters, epinephrine, and norepinephrine, which balance the more calming serotonin. Tyrosine therapies (targeted amino acids) are effective for fatigue symptoms, especially if you are using antidepressants, which may lower epinephrine or norepinephrine levels when increasing serotonin.

Other Adrenal Supports

Adrenal extracts are actual extracts of adrenal tissue obtained from pigs (porcine extract) or cows (bovine extract—most companies specify New Zealand bovine, since there are no mad cow disease possibilities from these sources). They contain adrenal nutrients as well as adrenal hormones and provide an effective remedy for low energy symptoms. I prescribe them frequently. Unlike horse estrogen (Premarin), the adrenal hormones in pigs and cows have the same structure as the hormones made by our bodies. Because adrenal hormones do not cause a rise in SHBG (sex hormone binding globulin), these extracts can be taken by mouth without the adverse effects in the liver that arise when taking oral sex hormones. They are available without a prescription and can be taken on an empty stomach. Because they contain many adrenal hormones, including aldosterone, they shouldn't be taken if your aldosterone is high, and they should be used cautiously if you have high blood pressure. Always let your doctor know if you are using adrenal extracts. They are potent.

Adrenal extracts should be taken like cortisol—first thing in the morning, again at noon, and if needed, later in the day around 3 or 4 p.m. Don't take too much adrenal support too late in the day because it will disturb your sleep. If you use too much, you may develop stomach upset, anxiety, palpitations, insomnia, or lower thyroid hormone levels.

Ginseng

Ginseng has been used for centuries by many cultures throughout the world. In China it is said to be able to "keep your virgin face younger and prolong your life forever and ever." Now, that sure beats Botox. There are many varieties of ginseng, and each has a slightly different property, but all fortify your immune system. Common ginsengs are listed here to help you decide which best suits you.

- **Siberian ginseng** (*Eleutherococcus senticosus*) is energizing and particularly good for physical stress. Athletes in training and adrenal-depleted walking wounded often use it.
- **Korean ginseng** (*Panax ginseng*) is similar to Siberian ginseng in that it is good for physical stress and it will improve exercise capacity. It is considered a sexual tonic in Asia, improving erectile function and libido.
- **Indian ginseng, ashwagandha** (*Withania somnifera*) is calming. It is useful if you have anxiety or insomnia; and oddly enough, it also helps if you have fatigue. It also supports thyroid hormone production of T4.

Other Herbs

- **Rhodiola** (*Rhodiola rosea*) is useful if you are under mental stress or overworked. It has been shown to support memory as well as physical stamina. Interestingly, low doses are energizing, but high doses can actually be relaxing and useful for anxiety symptoms.
- **Ginkgo** (*Ginkgo biloba*) is primarily known for its ability to improve blood flow to many organs, but it also helps the brain-adrenal connection (the HPA (hypothalamus-pituitary axis that controls adrenal function). With chronic stress, the HPA is often imbalanced and depleted, and ginkgo can help this.
- **Astragalus** (*Astralagus membranaceous*) is particularly helpful to support immune function. I often recommend its use in my adrenally challenged patients during flu season to boost their immunity.
- **Cordyceps** (*Cordyceps sinsensis*) and **rhemania** (*Rhemanis glutinosa*) are herbs that act to support adrenal hormone production.

They can be found in many over-the-counter herbal adrenal blends and Chinese kidney yin tonics in combination with other herbs and vitamins.

Vitamins and Minerals

Vitamin C is probably the most important vitamin to support cortisol levels, which may be one reason that high doses of vitamin C (1,500 to 2,000 mg/day) seem to improve cold symptoms. Vitamin C is essential for adrenal hormone production, so if you are under stress, increase your vitamin C intake. Most animals have an ability to convert blood sugar into vitamin C to help them to cope with prolonged stress. Humans can't do that; we have to get it from food or pills.

Other vitamins that are important for adrenal support are vitamin E (800 units/day); B vitamins, particularly vitamin B_6 (50 to 100 mg/day); pantothenic acid (500 mg two to three times a day); and PABA (para-aminobenzoic acid, 300 to 1,500 mg/day). High doses of PABA have been shown to be effective in treating some autoimmune diseases, such as scleroderma, lupus, and rheumatoid arthritis. If you are using it be careful, as very high doses can lower your vitamin D production or affect your liver. Always use PABA under a doctor's care.

Thyroid Hormone Support

Low thyroid hormone levels are due either to low production by the thyroid or to poor activation of T4 into the active form, T3. Finding the best way for you to support thyroid function depends on determining what is causing your problem and how severe your symptoms are. People sometimes fear that once they are started on thyroid hormone, it is a life sentence; but that's not always the case, unless you have persistent thyroid antibodies.

Thyroid hormones should be used if your TSH level is greater than 2 mU/ml and there are low thyroid signs and symptoms. Many physicians believe in only using T4 to treat low thyroid conditions and only when the TSH has risen out of the normal range. I feel strongly that you should not wait until your TSH rises out of range because even at the high end of the normal ranges, low thyroid function will adversely affect your heart, mind, mood, muscles, bowels, and nerves. Thyroid symptoms should be treated before they become severe.

Using Thyroid Hormones

I often recommend using natural thyroid extract, such as desiccated Armour thyroid, derived from pigs. It contains T3 and T4 as well as other thyroid nutrients, such as T1 and T2. The effects of T1 and T2 are not well understood, but T2 appears to help increase the metabolism of fat and muscle. You could also use synthetic T4 (Levoxyl or Synthroid) and add T3 (Cytomel), or have a compounding pharmacy make T4 and/or T3 for you in individualized doses. Whatever form you decide to use, there are a few things to know about taking thyroid hormones:

- Thyroid hormones should always be taken on an empty stomach and never with any form of calcium or iron, as these can interfere with how they are absorbed.
- Start with low doses (15 mg of Armour thyroid, 25 mcg of T4, or 1 to 5 mcg of T3) and gradually increase over weeks. (Doses below 5 mcg of T3 will need to be compounded by your pharmacist.) When thyroid hormone is low, adenaline or noradrenaline is often high to compensate. It takes two to three days to down-regulate adrenaline and adrenaline receptors. For this reason, increase thyroid slowly, to avoid feeling too racy or having heart palpitations. Most people can tell what dose is best for them. How you feel is the best test. If you feel calm and have good energy, you are sleeping well, and your bowels are normal, you are right on the right track. If you feel nervous or anxious, you may need to reduce your dose or increase the dose more slowly.
- T4 circulates in your body for many days; T3, on the other hand, lasts only hours. For this reason some people feel best when T3 is given two to three times per day. Alternatively, your dose can be compounded into a slow-release form.
- Armour thyroid may not be the best choice for you if tests show that you have a high-normal T4 and a low-normal T3, or T4 activation problems. In such cases, use only T3 in as low a dose as needed.

- Dosages vary with different thyroid medications:
  - T3 can be compounded into 1 to 10 mcg doses or prescribed as Cytomel (the lowest available dose is 5 mcg).
  - T4 is available in many prescription doses (Synthroid or Levoxyl) ranging from 25 mcg to 300 mcg and can, of course, be compounded into any dose. I generally use 25-mcg doses and slowly increase the dose each week until either my patient feels great or blood or urine tests show a good level (TSH between 1 and 2 IU/ml, with midrange T4 and T3).
  - Armour thyroid is a purified extract from pig thyroid glands. It is bioidentical to human thyroid. Its dosing is unique. One grain is 60 mg and contains 9 mcg of T3 and 38 mcg of T4. I like it because it contains T1, T2, and calcitonin. The exact roles of T1 and T2 are not fully understood, but they help in thyroid metabolism; and calcitonin helps maintain calcium in your bones. Occasionally I have a patient who develops a stomach upset with Armour thyroid. If this happens, ask your pharmacist about trying Naturethroid, which is the same as Armour thyroid but does not have propylene glycol and may be better tolerated.
  - Thyrolar is a synthetic combination of T3 and T4 for people who do not wish to take animal products. Doses of Thyrolar vary. I usually start with one-fourth grain, or 15 mg (3.1 mcg of T3 and 12.5 mcg of T4) and gradually increase it. Few people need more than one grain. Remember, with any thyroid dose containing T3, over time the dose will be gradually reduced as your body becomes able to convert T4 into T3 more efficiently. Usually you will know you are ready to reduce your T3 by following your TSH, which should start to fall as your thyroid is strengthened (see below).

TSH Response to Therapy

Within days of starting replacement, your mood, energy, anxiety, and sleep should improve. If no improvement occurs, your dose can be increased slowly over several days or weeks. People who need thyroid support notice a sense of well-being almost immediately when the correct dose is reached.

Over time your TSH levels should return to normal. Aim to keep your TSH between 1 and 2 mU/ml. Again, how you feel should guide the dose. If your TSH level falls below 1 mU/ml, this is a good sign that your body's thyroid activation or function has improved and your support can be lowered and gradually withdrawn.

If a patient has many signs and symptoms of low thyroid function but her TSH is normal, I will sometimes prescribe a very-low-dose thyroid hormone (because the TSH is not always working perfectly) as a trial, and see how well she feels on this.

The goal is always to treat the true underlying problem. So always measure and treat any low levels of minerals and/or adrenal hormones (iron, magnesium, DHEA, cortisol, iodine, selenium). When your TSH level falls, withdraw thyroid support slowly. Most patients remain free of symptoms once the underlying problems (adrenal or mineral problems) have been treated. If you have persistently high thyroid antibodies, you may never be able to stop thyroid support, but you can lower your dose once adrenal and mineral problems are corrected.

Diet and Herbal Supports for Thyroid Function

If you have low thyroid function by TSH testing and positive thyroid antibodies, you need thyroid hormone, but some supplements and changes in your diet can also help your thyroid to function better. Selenium (200 to 300 mcg/day) has been found to lower thyroid antibody levels in some people.

Because the conversion of T4 into T3 requires many minerals including magnesium, selenium, iron, iodine, and copper as well as vitamins A, B_2, B_6, B_{12}, and C, a diet rich in minerals and vitamins including red meat, seaweed, dark green leafy vegetables, and seafood is important. Certain foods, known as goitrogens, can actually block thyroid hormone production when eaten raw or to excess. Examples of goitrogenic foods are turnips, cabbage, mustard greens, soybeans, cauliflower, peanuts, pine nuts, millet, and cassava root. If you have thyroid problems, usually not more than one of these foods daily is recommended. Fermented soy (tempeh or miso) does not cause any problems and can be eaten freely. Generally soy should be limited to 30 to 60 mg a day (5 to 8 oz of soy milk contain 30 mg of soy isoflavones).

Tyrosine can be helpful because it is the amino acid that makes thyroid hormone (as well as dopamine and adrenaline). It is found in lentils, beans, peas, seafood, meat (particularly wild game), fish, whey protein, eggs, soy, and dairy. If it is taken as a supplement, take it in the morning (usually 500 to 1000 mg); it can be repeated in the early afternoon. However, it can be stimulating and may keep you awake if taken too late in the day. Take tyrosine on an empty stomach (or at least away from proteins) to maximize its absorption.

Minerals are important for normal function and activation of thyroid hormones. Iodine is tricky because too much can be as bad as too little. I recommend 150 to 500 mcg a day, but use a much higher dose if there is breast disease. Other helpful minerals are iron (60 to 120 mg/day), zinc (15 to 50 mg/day), selenium (200 to 400 mcg/day), and magnesium (aspartate, taurate, or glycinate forms are best, 300 to 500 mg/day). If you have low RBC magnesium, use 400 to 500 mg/day and take your magnesium with taurine (500 to 2,000 mg/day) to help your cells absorb the magnesium.

Taurine is an amino acid that helps "feed," or mineralize, red blood cells. If you have low iron or magnesium, it will help improve your body's response to treatment. Taurine also helps support sleep and won't cause morning drowsiness. It is best taken at bedtime on an empty stomach. It can promote better sleep by enhancing GABA (the same neurotransmitter Ativan and Valium work on). Usual doses of taurine are 1,000 to 3,000 mg per day.

Magnesium glycinate is a form of magnesium that enters blood cells easily. Other good forms of magnesium are magnesium oxide, magnesium aspartate, and, of course, taurate. **Magnesium citrate** can cause loose bowel movements, so it is a good treatment if you are prone to constipation but can cause diarrhea if overused.

Bladderwrack is a type of seaweed that is added to many thyroid supplements to help T4 convert into T3. If you use it, or use products containing it, be careful not to use T3 (or use T3 with caution), as too much T3 can be formed. This can suppress your own thyroid hormone production. Signs of too much T3 are anxiety, excess energy, sleep disturbance, or palpitations. If this happens, reduce the bladderwrack and/or T3.

Julie: Perimenopause Cured with Thyroid and Adrenal Support

Julie was a fifty-two-year-old married mother of two teenagers, juggling her career and motherhood while trying to return to school and manage a singing group "for fun." She always had to push to get things done, but this was getting harder and harder to do. Reliable sleep, energy, and a stable mood had become things of the past.

When I met her she was still menstruating, but she had noticed that her previously regular periods were now happening every twenty-one days instead of every twenty-eight. Also, her menstrual bleeding, which had always been normal, was heavier and lasted seven days instead of three or four. The way she bled had changed, too. Usually she bled for a few days and it was over. Now she would spot for a couple of days, then it was as if gates opened and she had to change her tampons and pads every two hours, after which she would spot for more days. Headaches, which had never been a problem, were now occurring regularly during her menstrual cycles. She also had breast tenderness a few days before her periods, but she just assumed that was normal.

Julie's sleep was bad, especially before her period. She could fall asleep most nights, but found herself waking nearly every night at 3 a.m., and then she couldn't fall back to sleep until around 6:30 a.m., when she felt she could sleep all day. Her sleep felt too light, not restful, and she no longer dreamed. Her poor sleep made it hard to get going in the morning and her motivation in general was low. She became irritable and moody, and was easily brought to tears. Her memory and concentration were poor, and her sex drive was nearly nonexistent. She had vaginal dryness, making sex with her younger husband uncomfortable, even with over-the-counter lubricants.

When I examined Julie, I saw that her skin and hair were dry, she had lost much of her arm and leg hair (even her pubic hair was thinning), and her face looked tired and washed-out—all signs of low DHEA.

Julie was exhibiting the classic symptoms of perimenopause. Her erratic, at times heavy, menstrual bleeds with PMS, insomnia, and breast tenderness in the days or weeks before her period were all signs of progesterone deficiency. Her lack of sex drive, vaginal dryness, menstrual headaches, tearfulness, and draggy blah feelings with a lack of motivation during her periods were all typical signs of low estradiol. She also had many signs and symptoms of DHEA deficiency: irritable mood, loss of memory, low sex drive, light sleep without dreams, dry skin, and loss of body hair. Her low energy and weak pulses (a sign of weak kidneys in Chinese medicine) painted a low adrenal picture.

Her blood and twenty-four-hour urine tests revealed that everything was normal to the untrained eye. Normal, yes, but well below the midrange, and certainly not normal for her. Blood tests showed her DHEA-S was barely in the low range of normal, more what you would expect of a woman in her seventies or eighties (a distinction not made by adult DHEA normal ranges). Her iron and magnesium were also low, most likely from all of the heavy bleeding, and her estradiol was low (48 pg/ml). Some doctors would consider this normal, but I have found that most women feel best when their estradiol is over 60 pg/ml. In a menopausal woman there is no "normal" range, but I aim to support the estradiol level at a range of about 60 to 80 pg/ml. Julie's twenty-four-hour urine test showed a low aldosterone, low-normal cortisol, and a very-low-normal DHEA. Her thyroid levels on both the blood and urine tests were fine.

At the first visit I started Julie on progesterone. Because she had trouble sleeping and had very heavy periods, I chose oral natural progesterone. It would help her sleep and is reliably absorbed. Because her periods were so heavy, I also prescribed progesterone cream during the day to ensure a good level of progesterone throughout the day. She took two 100 mg progesterone capsules at bedtime and applied 100 mg of progesterone cream to her abdomen and breasts in the morning. (If she had been overweight, I would have told her to apply the cream to her inner and outer arm.)

To support her adrenal glands, I started her on 5 mg of DHEA in the morning with 5 mg of pregnenolone, and an adrenal extract in the morning and at noon. (I used an adrenal extract because it contains some cortisol and some aldosterone. Ginseng would support cortisol, but not her aldosterone. She could have used ginseng and licorice root, which has an aldosterone-like effect, instead of the extract.) I did not prescribe estradiol at this time, because it might have worsened her breast tenderness and heavy bleeding, but I explained to her that if she improved the breakdown of estrogen in her liver, many of her liver symptoms (such as headaches, breast tenderness, and irritability) would likely improve. She agreed to stop drinking coffee and improve her diet by eating more cruciferous vegetables high in I3C (indole-3-carbinol). She also started taking flax meal (ground flaxseeds) every day. I explained to her that treating her adrenal glands, particularly her DHEA, would help support her estrogen indirectly and perhaps improve her mood, sleep, sex drive, and stamina. I gave her a list of estrogen-deficient symptoms (listed in appendix A) and told her to contact me if these symptoms didn't improve on this regimen.

Julie did very well—so well that she didn't come back for four months. She began cycling regularly at twenty-eight-day intervals on the progesterone, and her bleeding, though still heavy, was less and she now bled for only four days. Her sleep was great so long as she took her progesterone. Without it she woke at 3 a.m. and had trouble falling back to sleep. Her mood was better and she was less irritable, but she still had a tendency to the blues. Her headaches were also better, but she still had a little headache during her menstrual cycle and she still had a very low sex drive.

At her four-month visit we reviewed her labs and discussed her low minerals, particularly her low iron and magnesium. I have found that it is nearly impossible to reduce heavy bleeding in a patient with persistently low levels of iron. According to Chinese medicine, the blood is too thin when it is anemic, and it flows like water. So I started Julie on iron (ferrous sulfate, 100 mg/day) in addition to taurine (3,000 mg/day) with magnesium glycinate (500 mg/day).

Four months into her treatment, we decided to add estradiol, cautiously, to see if it would improve her low sex drive, palpitations, and persistent (though improved) headaches and low moods, without causing breast tenderness or heavier bleeding. I prescribed estradiol lotion (1 mg/ml) with instructions to use 0.3 to 0.5 ml twice daily, applied to her inner and outer arm. I explained to her how she could control her own dosages to address her symptoms. She should reduce the dose if she had any vaginal spotting or breast tenderness, and she should increase the estradiol dose if she had menstrual headaches or felt particularly blue during her period (when estradiol is lowest in the cycle). I also increased her DHEA from 5 to 10 mg (in the morning) since her levels had been so low and I knew that this would further support her sex hormones while providing more energy. She continued taking her adrenal extract and 5 mg of pregnenolone.

On this new regimen her mood became more level and her sex drive returned. She no longer had vaginal dryness or dry eyes. Her sleep was deeper and she slept through the night. She did notice, however, that if she stopped her DHEA, her sleep was not as good—it was less deep and restful. Her cycles gradually improved. Each cycle became less heavy and occurred regularly every twenty-eight days, without PMS, breast tenderness, or insomnia.

In the following months, she did so well that she stopped using oral progesterone and simply used progesterone cream morning and night on days 15 to 25 of her cycle. She continued her estradiol (regularly using 0.4 ml twice daily on days 1 to 25 of the cycle). On this regimen she remained headache-free with normal cycles, good energy, stable mood, and a good sex drive free of vaginal dryness. As an added bonus, she reported fewer colds and flu (DHEA is an important support for the immune system).

Julie now sees me twice a year to measure her DHEA-S and follow her magnesium and iron levels in her blood. She also does a yearly twenty-four-hour urine test to monitor how well her body is metabolizing her estrogen, progesterone, and DHEA hormones.

Jane: When Cortisol Pays the Price for Missed Perimenopause

Jane's therapist referred her to me to see if I could do anything for her poor sleep and terrible fatigue. No one had ever treated these problems successfully, and Jane wasn't even sure that she wanted to waste her time on me, but she was willing to try anything. She had many medical problems and symptoms such as depression, reflux, high blood pressure, and unusual chest pains. Jane had seen multiple doctors and had many tests done, only to be told, "We don't know what these chest pains are, but they don't seem to be serious."

She had been on disability for one and a half years for severe, incapacitating nerve pains in her legs and chronic low back pains, which were only relieved by nerve blocks every three to six months. To make matters worse, she had gained over thirty pounds in two years.

All of Jane's symptoms had started in her early forties, when she began having heavy, painful, and irregular periods. Unfortunately for her, this common perimenopausal problem was never treated with progesterone. As her menstrual problems worsened, so did her sleep.

By age forty-nine she was not sleeping, was growing large uterine fibroids, and having uncontrolled, heavy, erratic bleeding and terrible fatigue. Eventually, at the age of fifty-one, she required a hysterectomy and both of her ovaries were removed. This relieved her heavy bleeding, but not her sleep or energy problems. Following surgery Jane refused hormone replacement, like so many women scared by the WHI study, and her sleep problems only intensified. When she was finally able to fall asleep, it felt too light and unrefreshing. She usually woke prematurely in the early morning around 4 a.m. Jane's insomnia was most likely a symptom of progesterone deficiency. Perhaps progesterone begun early enough would have spared Jane her hysterectomy.

The extent of her fatigue was daunting. She was no longer able to do the things she had loved. Prior to her disability, she had worked full-time and had taken care of the house and even her husband's business. Now she struggled to get through her day, not working, not doing housework. It was all terribly depressing for her. Even when she had relief from her pains with pain-blocking injections, she couldn't enjoy herself.

Whenever I hear someone describe such debilitating fatigue, I usually find a problem with adrenal function. I questioned her about symptoms of low cortisol and low DHEA. Sure enough, despite her weight gain, she had no appetite. In fact, she felt nauseated much of the time, which is commonly seen with cortisol deficiency. She was prone to irritability if stressed or pressured, and at times she felt lightheaded. Her memory was poor and she had no sex drive.

She had had her thyroid tested and had been told that "everything is okay," but she had many symptoms of low thyroid function, such as thinning hair, dry skin, memory loss, always feeling cold, and bruising easily. In addition, she couldn't seem to lose weight, no matter what diet she tried. She was moody and depressed, and her bowels were erratic.

When I examined her, I saw that she was overweight (five feet tall and 286 pounds), with thinning hair on her scalp. She had very dry skin with thick calluses on her heels, and her reflexes were sluggish—all common physical signs of poor thyroid function. Further, she had relatively no body hair, thinning pubic hair, and the dry hair typically seen in women with low DHEA.

I ordered blood tests and a twenty-four-hour urine test. She still chose not to use any estrogen or progesterone, but she was happy to try some adrenal and thyroid support while awaiting her test results. I started her on a low dose of thyroid hormone (using only T4, 25 mcg/day) and after a couple of days added a low dose of cortisol (5 mg in the morning and 2.5 mg at noon) with DHEA (10 mg in the morning). If her energy was still low, I told her to add a small dose of pregnenolone (5 mg).

After she started her new regimen, the results of her blood tests and twenty-four-hour urine tests came back. They showed very low levels of cortisol and DHEA. Her thyroid levels showed T4 and T3 levels that, although normal, were well below midrange. Her blood tests were within normal ranges, but all hormone levels were well below the midrange. Her pregnenolone and DHEA-S levels were below normal ranges. I increased her cortisol to 10 mg in the morning and continued 5 mg at noon. I also increased her DHEA to 30 mg for two months, with a gradually lowered dose after this when I added a low dose of T3 (5 mcg).

On this regimen Jane began to have almost normal energy and was able to do daily activities. Her atypical chest pains stopped completely. Following these adjustments she was able to sleep for six hours through the night and she fell back to sleep more easily when she woke. Her bowels slowly improved, and she was able to lose twelve pounds. Though she still suffers from her underlying nerve pains, the overall improvement in her life has been remarkable. She has continued on adrenal supports and amino acid therapies to support her epinephrine and serotonin levels. She has regained a life; and even without using sex hormones, she is a happier person.

11

Sleep Hormones

Good sleep comes on effortlessly, lasts solidly through the night with pleasant dreams, and finds you waking six to eight hours later feeling refreshed. "Hah," you may be thinking, "I haven't had that in years, if ever." Well, it is attainable. Sleep is affected by many factors—environmental, physical, and emotional. Some things you can control, like what you eat and do before bed or what time you go to bed. Others you may not be able to alter, such as your neighbor's music or loud noises in the night. These things aside, there are two hormones that can help you attain restful, refreshing sleep: melatonin and growth hormone. I consider both of these hormones at the final stages of any hormone restoration project. Think of them as the finishing touches to your hormone makeover, improving any remaining symptoms not improved by sex, adrenal, or thyroid hormones.

It may seem odd to lump these two hormones together, as they are vastly different and do not have much interaction with each other (although melatonin can raise growth hormone levels). Melatonin is inexpensive and available at any pharmacy or health food store. Growth hormone, on the other hand, is expensive, controversial, and not easy to come by. Both are difficult to measure, and when either is chronically low, you will sleep poorly, age prematurely, and feel more anxious about things.

Both melatonin and growth hormone decline as you age, but for some reason melatonin falls at a greater rate around the time of peri-menopause, often worsening already poor sleep due to a lack of pro-gesterone. Because growth hormone is primarily produced during the dreaming phase of sleep, growth hormone deficiency often follows and accompanies melatonin deficiency.

Not everyone needs these hormones. In fact, if your sleep is solid and refreshing, you may not even need to read this chapter (unless you want to learn how melatonin helps jet lag and the winter blues). I estimate that about 75 percent of my patients stop their hormone program at the end of chapter 10. Once sex hormones are balanced (by normal levels of thyroid and adrenal hormones), most people feel better than ever and are usually sleeping well. This chapter is for shift workers, night owls, anti-aging enthusiasts, and the remaining minority who, though they generally have good energy and stable moods, are still not sleeping through the night. For them a good night's sleep is elusive. Here's how to get it with melatonin. Chapter 12 discusses growth hormone.

Good Sleep

We all need a good night's sleep for a stable mood, a good memory, and a strong immune system. Sleep is mysterious. It occurs in repeating ninety-minute cycles, controlled by your inner clock (regulated by melatonin). Each sleep cycle contains five stages of sleep. Each stage of sleep varies in duration as the night proceeds. The first two stages of sleep are lighter than the later stages and, as the night progresses, these light and deep stages shorten and dream states—REM (rapid eye movement)—expand. Gradually, more time is spent in REM sleep. REM is a truly restorative time for your body and as we age, the amount of time spent in REM, restorative, delta-wave sleep lessens.

The first two stages are light sleep. During this time, people are sensitive to noises and easily awakened. Not a lot happens in these early stages of sleep other than slowing your thoughts, heart rate, and breathing, and relaxing your muscles. The really great parts of sleep happen in the deep stages (stages three and four) and in the final stage, REM sleep. REM sleep is a light sleep and leads to waking. During deep sleep the body is restored, cells are repaired, and healing takes place. During REM sleep we dream; our neurotransmitters, which control our emotions, are replenished; and memories are made (short-term memory is transferred to parts of the brain to become long-term memories). Good sleep is sleep that has enough deep and REM stages. REM sleep is most important. If we are wakened during a REM cycle, our sleep cycle is changed and the next time we sleep we will go almost directly back into REM to complete its magic. Without good sleep we become moody, have difficulty concentrating, become hormonally imbalanced, undergo neurotransmitter depletion, and suffer memory loss. Most sleep medications shorten the amount of time necessary to reach deep sleep but almost all cause a shortening of both deep and REM sleep. For this reason they are not recommended for long-term use. Trazadone is one of the few medications that does not seem to affect this, and this rather weak antidepressant is often used to treat long-term sleep disturbance.

Our ninety-minute sleep cycles usually repeat three to five times per night. Melatonin helps our sleep by increasing both deep and REM phases of sleep. Melatonin ensures that as the night continues, the time spent in deep and REM sleep progressively increases. As morning approaches, our sleep becomes deeper and more dream-filled, and with this we feel refreshed and renewed.

Bad Sleep

As we age, our melatonin falls, and the amounts of deep sleep and REM phases of sleep also decline. This can be a problem because growth hormone is primarily produced during the deep phases of sleep, and our old neurotransmitters are discharged and new ones are regenerated during REM sleep. The brain is sort of like a battery that must be discharged before it can be fully recharged. Our dreams are largely the result of high levels of neurotransmitters discharging. So if you are having bad sleep, know that your body probably isn't making enough growth hormone or restoring neurotransmitters optimally.

Most people start to notice a deterioration in the quality of their sleep in their mid-forties. Certainly by age fifty, most notice that their sleep is more easily disturbed, less dream-filled, and not as refreshing as it used to be. Lifestyles with a lot of late-night activities, bright night lights, late meals, and excess caffeine and alcohol further deplete our dwindling middle-aged melatonin reserves and worsen our sleep problems.

Sleep disorders are common. Sixty-two percent of Americans have some type of sleep problem, and more than 35 million Americans suffer from long-term insomnia. Chronic insomnia can lead to a problem with your immune system, and can cause or worsen growth hormone deficiency as well as adrenal fatigue and premature aging. Bad sleep increases your chances of heart disease and obesity. Without enough REM sleep, we become forgetful, irritable, and depressed. Unfortunately, while many of the sleeping pills that we use are sedating, they do not increase our deficient REM and deep-sleep cycles.

If you are using hormone supports and you are not sleeping well, make sure that your hormone plan is balanced. You should have enough progesterone to balance your estrogen. Your DHEA should not be too low or too high. You shouldn't be taking too much adrenal support, and your adrenal supports shouldn't be taken too late in the day (after 3 p.m.). Make sure that you are absorbing sex hormone creams (check a blood test to ensure that the hormone creams are being well absorbed), and ensure that your thyroid hormone is optimal, but not excessive. If all of these things are okay and your sleep is still not sound, then you should measure your nighttime melatonin, cortisol, and growth hormone. While waiting for your results, give melatonin a try. Don't even think about trying growth hormone until you know that you need it.

What Melatonin Does for You

Melatonin is the hormone of hibernation in animals and is produced in a tiny region of the human brain known as the pineal gland. Melatonin does all the things you would want to do if you were hibernating—it relaxes you, makes you sleepy, cools your body, and lets you sleep while entertaining you with interesting dreams. It is the only hormone affected by light, temperature, and electromagnetic fields.

Melatonin controls the deep and dream phases of your sleep. When your melatonin is low, your sleep is light, you are easily awakened, and you have few, if any, dreams. You may have difficulty falling asleep, and usually there is a real problem falling back to sleep once you are awake. Typically, if your melatonin is low, you will find yourself waking with an anxious feeling in the middle of the night for no good reason. When melatonin is chronically low, people age prematurely, have a lack of ambition, and move more slowly than usual during the day. Concentration and recall are poor, and depression is common.

Although melatonin is primarily the hormone of sleep, it does many other things. It is a potent antioxidant, supports the immune system, improves the activation of thyroid hormone by making T3, and increases the levels of all of your sex hormones, as well as growth hormone. It lowers cortisol levels and can reduce the effects of estrogen, too.

Melatonin is used to treat insomnia, jet lag, cancer (studies have shown a role for melatonin in breast cancer, as it seems to block estrogen from binding to estrogen receptors), depression, hypertension (melatonin can lower systolic blood pressure), and seasonal affective disorder (SAD). The symptoms of SAD are irritability, fatigue, low mood, weight gain, and carbohydrate cravings, and all of these symptoms tend to be worse in winter months.

How Melatonin Is Made

Melatonin is made from serotonin. Depression is often due to low serotonin levels. When serotonin levels are low, melatonin levels may also be low. This explains why sleep disturbance often accompanies depression, particularly during menopause, when estradiol is no longer able to fully support serotonin levels. Optimim melatonin production depends on many things. It is produced from the amino acid tryptophan and requires a fancy methylation process involving methionine and SAMe, as well as B vitamins (particularly B_{12} and B_6) and N-acetylcysteine (NAC).

Understanding how melatonin is made is important because some people are sensitive to it and have trouble using it. Such people can improve their melatonin levels by taking its component parts: tryptophan, methionine, NAC, SAMe, and vitamins B_{12} and B_6.

How Melatonin Works

Once melatonin is made, it must be activated. Your sleeping environment holds the key. Darkness activates melatonin; light suppresses it. The activation of melatonin by darkness helps to regulate your circadian rhythm, the internal clock that makes you sleepy at night and awake during the day. Melatonin is activated gradually, beginning after sunset and peaking between 11 p.m. and 2 a.m. That is why it is best to fall asleep as melatonin is rising, say, from 11 to 1 a.m., to get its full effect. Going to bed later than 1 a.m. is usually not as refreshing, since melatonin levels are lower. When daylight approaches, melatonin will be suppressed. Daytime sleep is usually not as restorative because there is little or no melatonin to support your deep and REM stages of sleep. In the winter months, when days are shortest, melatonin levels are highest, because there is less light to suppress it. This can make people feel lethargic and lazy and want to eat—in effect, to prepare for hibernation.

Circadian rhythms vary from individual to individual. Most people's internal clock is around twenty-four hours, coinciding with the amount of time it takes for Earth to rotate on its axis. Early birds, who naturally like to rise early, have a short clock, less than twenty-four hours. Night owls, who like to stay up late, have an internal clock closer to twenty-six hours. Lifestyles that involve late nights, frequent travel, late meals, late-night alcohol, late-night computer work, nighttime exercise, and excessive night stimulation tend to foster lower melatonin levels, which reinforces night owl behavior.

Measuring Melatonin

If you want to be scientific about your sleep, you can measure your melatonin level, but I usually use melatonin tests only when I'm stumped, since a trial of melatonin is easy, cheap, and quick. If you are checking melatonin levels, I usually recommend checking nighttime cortisol as well, if you have a resistant insomnia problem. Melatonin only stays around in your system for a short time and is mainly produced in the middle of the night, so the best way to measure melatonin is from a saliva test done in the middle of the night, when you are waking spontaneously or can't fall asleep. I find these spit tests helpful, although critics question their reliability. Urine tests for melatonin metabolites may be more reliable. These tests have recently become available with some labs in this country.

Diet and Melatonin

Some bedtime snacks can help melatonin production in the brain. Melatonin is made from the amino acid tryptophan, but in order to get tryptophan from your food into your brain cells, you need insulin (stimulated by carbohydrates). Insulin selectively pushes tryptophan into your brain cells. For these reasons, just eating protein (high in tryptophan) alone doesn't have the same calming effect because proteins contain other amino acids that can be stimulating and defeat the calming tryptophan effect. Eating plain carbohydrates alone (to get the necessary insulin) also doesn't work, as these are often too stimulating. The best foods for sleep are dairy, bananas, oats, sweet corn, rice, tomatoes, and whey protein. The home remedy of warm milk at bedtime is, in fact, grounded in science.

Drugs and Melatonin

Many recreational drugs and medications affect melatonin and contribute to sleep problems.

Marijuana raises melatonin levels more dramatically than any other drug. Its effect typically occurs almost immediately (within twenty minutes of smoking) and results in very high levels (as much as four thousand times the normal baseline). Such high levels can cause rebound insomnia (see melatonin overdose below) and can deplete melatonin or tryptophan levels, resulting in disturbed, unrefreshing sleep and moodiness. If marijuana is used during the day, when melatonin is normally not made, a phase shift in the natural circadian rhythm can occur, resulting in sleepiness during the day and wakefulness at night.

Caffeine, the nicotine in tobacco, and alcohol all lower melatonin levels. Alcohol inhibits melatonin production and also suppresses REM sleep as well as the deepest phase of sleep, the delta phase. Any of these consumed within an hour of bedtime reduces melatonin by about one half, which may delay sleep from starting or may disrupt the later restorative phases of sleep.

Many medications affect melatonin levels. These are listed at the end of this chapter.

Improve Your Melatonin Level and Your Sleep

1. Lowering your body temperature helps melatonin. Taking a hot bath one or two hours before bed will raise your body temperature. When you get out of the tub, the fall in temperature supports melatonin production. (A hot shower does not raise your body temperature as much as a hot bath does.)
2. Stress and worry reduce melatonin production. Find ways to relax before going to bed. Relaxation tapes, yoga, and meditation can improve melatonin production.
3. Strenuous mental activity should be stopped at least one hour before bedtime
4. Bright lights at night reduce melatonin. Use a low-watt nightlight if you get up in the middle of the night.
5. Go to bed before 1 a.m. because melatonin production peaks before 2 a.m. If you habitually go to bed later than this, slowly work to reset your internal clock by rising slightly earlier and retiring slightly earlier each day.
6. Overeating lowers melatonin, lack of food stimulates it. If you are going to have a large dinner, finish at least four hours before bedtime.
7. Avoid consuming alcohol four to five hours before bedtime.
8. Avoid caffeine four to six hours before bedtime.
9. Going to bed and waking up in a routine way each day, as close

to light/dark cues as possible, ensures the most stable circadian rhythm, which in turn provides optimal melatonin.

10. Foods containing tryptophan and complex carbohydrates help melatonin. Whey protein, bananas, or dairy snacks at bedtime can be helpful.

11. Vitamins B_{12} and B_6 are needed to make melatonin, and vitamin B_3 (niacin) prevents breakdown of tryptophan. A vitamin B complex formula (50 to 100 mg/day), taken any time of day, can be helpful to support melatonin production.

12. Other nutrients that help your body make melatonin are NAC (500 to 1000 mg), methionine (500 to 1000 mg) taken in the morning, and tryptophan (100 to 200) of 5-HTP (5-hydroxytrp-tophan, 50 to 100 mg) taken at bedtime.

13. Calcium at bedtime can increase melatonin production.

14. Regular exercise helps melatonin production, but it will inhibit melatonin if done too late in the day. Avoid exercising within three to four hours of bedtime.

15. Exposure to sunlight for at least twenty minutes each morning ensures that your internal clock is properly signaled to delay melatonin production. This is especially important in winter months.

How to Take Melatonin

If you've tried melatonin and it didn't work, then you probably used the wrong dose. Odd as it may seem, it is often the case that the lower the dose, the more potent the effect. This is counterintuitive; if you take melatonin and sleep is not improved, try a lower dose.

The correct dose of melatonin varies from individual to individual, regardless of size or sex. For example, I am very sensitive to it and can only use 0.1 mg per day. More than that, and the next morning I will have a headache with a groggy, hungover feeling. Most people do well on doses between 0.5 and 1 mg. Although melatonin is available in most drugstores in tablets, capsules, or sublingual forms, most preparations come in doses that are too high (3 to 5 mg). There is also a great variation in quality. How medications or supplements are prepared can affect how much is actually absorbed into your body. This is known as bioavailability. Pharmaceutical-grade products ensure proper bioavailability. That is, the substance can be used by the body at the dose stated. Many supplements differ in price depending upon their bioavailability. Some products seem like a better deal, but your body may be able to absorb only a portion of the supplement.

If melatonin never worked for you and/or you are having melatonin-deficient symptoms, you may want to ask a compounding pharmacist to make a dose of 0.1 mg and gradually increase the dose by 0.1 mg every two to three nights until your sleep is deep and restful. Many people have problems absorbing melatonin from their stomach and do better with a sublingual dose (a lozenge or a tablet that dissolves under the tongue). Sublingual doses get the melatonin directly into your bloodstream. They work faster than pills and usually have a stronger effect (that is, if you normally use 1 mg of oral melatonin, you may need only 0.5 mg of a sublingual dose).

The timing of the dose is also important. Usually an oral dose should be taken thirty to sixty minutes before bedtime. A sublingual dose is best taken fifteen minutes before bedtime. However, some people find that using melatonin an hour or two before bedtime works better; they fall asleep easier and have less of a drugged feeling in the morning. Dosing often requires a bit of trial and error.

Melatonin Overdose

If the dose of melatonin is too high, you may experience some of these side effects:

- Waking in the middle of the night, with difficulty falling back to sleep
- Palpitations or anxious feelings (often due to excess thyroid, T3 conversion)
- Disturbing, vivid dreams
- Headaches, or a feeling that your head is too big
- Groggy or hungover feelings in the morning

If any of these occur, lower the dose by one half. Not everyone can tolerate melatonin. So if a half dose doesn't work, stop taking it. Instead, try methionine (500 to 1,000 mg) in the morning on an empty stomach, with NAC (N-acetylcysteine, 600 mg twice daily) and B complex (100 mg) during meals to help methylate the methionine. In addition, use tryptophan (100 to 200 mg) at bedtime or as a targeted amino acid therapy with 5-HTP (5-hydroxytryptophan, 50 to 100 mg).

Kathy: Sleepless in Boston

Kathy was fifty years old, a working mother who had been doing pretty well with her sleep since starting estradiol and progesterone creams. Things would be okay until she had a presentation at work—then her sleep would become nearly impossible. She could usually fall asleep without any problem, but she would be up at 3 or 4 a.m., and no matter what she did she couldn't get back to sleep.

I checked a nighttime saliva test, taken at 4 a.m. when she woke spontaneously. Her melatonin was low and her cortisol was high. I thought she would be an easy fix. I recommended melatonin (0.5 mg) an hour before bed, and told her that if that didn't work, increase it to 1 mg. In addition, I prescribed phosphatidylserine (100 mg three times daily with meals) to help regulate her cortisol.

The first night she slept deeper, but felt drugged and headachy. She decided to see what a double dose would be like the next night. On this she had horrible dreams about demons and blood and woke feeling even more drugged and hung over than the previous day. Needless to say, she stopped everything and was discouraged.

She was clearly not tolerating melatonin, even though she had used it successfully in the past for jet lag. I explained to her that I would give her the building blocks to make melatonin herself. She started methionine (1,000 mg) in the morning before breakfast, and she took B complex (100 mg) and NAC (600 mg) with her breakfast and lunch. At bedtime she took three capsules of phosphatidylserine (100 mg each) to lower her high nighttime cortisol, with tryptophan (200 mg). Her sleep deepened almost immediately, and she gradually started sleeping normally. Interestingly, after a few months, she was able to tolerate melatonin 1 mg without side effects and she slowly withdrew the other supports.

Caution: Dangerous Interactions with Melatonin

Melatonin by itself is safe and effective, but there are some interactions to be aware of. It should not be used if you are pregnant or breast-feeding. Melatonin may increase the risk of bleeding in patients on warfarin (Coumadin), so you will need to consult your doctor before using it. Melatonin will lower steroid (cortisol) effects and the effects of the blood pressure medication clonidine. Some animal studies have shown that melatonin may lower the antidepressant effect of desipramine (Norpramin) and fluoxetine (Prozac). But fluoxetine itself lowers melatonin levels and may be one reason sleep can be a problem with its use.

Jet Lag

Melatonin works great for jet lag, both upon arrival and upon return from your destination. When you arrive, take melatonin one to three hours before your desired bedtime for three nights, and do the same when you return home. If you are on melatonin regularly, double your dose for these nights, then return to your usual dose after about three days. If you don't usually use it and don't know what dose to use, 1 to 2 mg per day typically works well. Make sure you buy a tablet that you can break, so if the dose is too high, you can lower it. I generally recommend traveling with 0.5 mg doses for this reason.

I also recommend using adrenal supports in the morning and afternoon to improve your energy for the first two to three days of travel. Much of the jet-lag feeling of fatigue is due to insufficient cortisol during the daytime. If you are taking regular adrenal support, double the morning dose for three days on either end of the trip, and you should be fine. I often prescribe adrenal extracts or natural hydrocortisone (Cortef), 10 mg in the morning and 5 mg at noon for three days on either end of the trip.

Seasonal Affective Disorder

During winter months, prolonged winter darkness causes increased melatonin production during the day. High daytime melatonin can cause SAD (seasonal affective disorder), characterized by fatigue, depression, weight gain, and carbohydrate cravings. Exposure to very bright light (even low-intensity light from indoor fluorescent lighting), particularly early in the morning and/or throughout the day, can prevent melatonin release and lift the mood and energy. If you are sleepy too early during winter nights, expose yourself to bright light in the late afternoon or evening, as this will delay melatonin production.

Interestingly enough, SAD is more common in people new to a northern region than in natives. Depressive symptoms last longer the farther north one lives.

Delayed Sleep Phase Insomnia and Rebound Insomnia

Night owl behavior may not be a problem, but it can lead to delayed sleep phase insomnia, which can be difficult to treat. People with this type of insomnia find themselves staying up later and later; and when they do sleep during light/waking hours, the sleep is not refreshing. They find it hard to fall asleep at normal times, usually because they are out of sync with normal light-and-dark cues for adequate melatonin production and most have also lost normal cortisol rhythms (see chapter 10). They are in a perpetually jet-lagged state, with cortisol rising late in the day instead of first thing in the morning. Sleeping pills only make the problem worse because many sleep aids shorten both deep and REM phases of sleep.

In order to treat delayed sleep insomnia effectively, you have to shift your sleep cycles back to normal rhythms. To do this, try bright light exposure early in the day for about twenty minutes and take melatonin in the hours before bedtime. Gradually shifting your bedtime to take advantage of melatonin's natural 11 p.m. to 2 a.m. peak will also help greatly. Often people need to use cortisol (5 to 10 mg) in the morning with phosphoserine (300 to 500 mg) taken in divided doses throughout the day and at bedtime to help lower afternoon/evening cortisol levels. Melatonin taken an hour before your anticipated bedtime can also help.

Drugs and Supplements That
Lower Melatonin

- Beta-blockers: propranolol (Inderal), atenolol (Tenormin), metoprolol (Lopressor, Toprol)
- Benzodiazepines: diazepam (Valium), alproazolam (Xanax), triazolam
- Calcium channel blockers: nifedipine (Adalat), verapamil (Isoptin)
- Antihypertensives: clonidine
- Anti-inflammatories: ibuprofen or aspirin
- Lithium
- Antidepressants: fluoxetine (Prozac)
- Tranquilizers
- Caffeine
- Tobacco
- Excess cortisol

12

Growth Hormone

From chapter 11, you know that normal levels of growth hormone are essential for deep, refreshing sleep. It is also important for calm and stable moods and it helps to burn fat and build muscles and bones. Studies have shown that growth hormone reduces obesity and heart disease, improves memory and immune function, and supports sex hormone production. When I first mention growth hormone to my patients, they almost always ask, "Why do I need that, I'm no longer growing?" But growth hormone has been hailed by many as the major anti-aging hormone, able to turn back the clock.

Growth hormone is a protein-based hormone produced by the pituitary gland primarily while you sleep. During our first twenty years of life, its levels are high and necessary to ensure that you reach your full height. Our growth hormone levels begin to fall as early as our twenties and continue to fall as we age. Loss of growth hormone is believed to be partly responsible for many of the signs and symptoms that we associate with aging.

Unfortunately, the first growth hormone available was obtained from human cadavers, and in the early years of therapy many growth hormone deficient–children contracted the equivalent of mad cow disease from injections of growth hormone from such sources. In the mid-1980s, bioidentical growth hormone was produced from recombinant DNA technology. Now safe, yet expensive, growth hormone is available by injection only. After its discovery in 1958, growth hormone was initially used only in children who failed to grow. But in 1990, a landmark study published in the *New England Journal of Medicine* showed that growth hormone injections given to men aged sixty one to eighty-one produced an improved sense of well-being, better muscle mass, and improved lean body mass (they lost weight in all the right places). It was claimed that growth hormone injections had reversed their aging by ten to twenty years. This was the beginning of the growth hormone craze, and treatments with growth hormone to prevent or reverse the effects of aging on skin, bone, mind, and spirit became popular.

Low Growth Hormone

People with low growth hormone can look and feel tired and old. Unlike adrenal fatigue that is worse in the afternoon, or thyroid fatigue that is worse in the morning, growth hormone fatigue is constant. You're just bone-tired all day long. People with low growth hormone feel even more tired if they stay out too late or do too much. I call this "payback fatigue." If you have even a little too much fun, there is a payback of exhaustion the next day.

People with low growth hormone are anxious, but they aren't really aware of their anxiety, they are just easily overwhelmed. Everyday problems seem too difficult to manage. A victimized type of anxiety is typical. They have a "Why me?" or "Oh, no, not again!" feeling when things go wrong. The world is against them. These people are reactive, not proactive, constantly putting out fires. Once growth hormone is normalized, there is a sense of well-being and people become more confident and positive. Everyday problems are just that—not the end of the world, simply problems to be dealt with. People become leaders. They become masters of their own universe.

If growth hormone is low, then sleep is poor, which only adds to the problem, since most growth hormone is produced during the deepest phases of sleep (phases 3 and 4), which lessen as we age. When you are low in growth hormone, sleep feels light and is easily interrupted. Sleep doesn't feel refreshing, and you have the sense that you have been up all night even though your bed partner may say that you seemed to sleep enough.

The physical signs of growth hormone deficiency keep plastic surgeons busy. Facial lines or creases deepen. Lips become thin, less full. Just look at the lips of any elderly person—the upper lip is nearly nonexistent. Because growth hormone builds muscle, the muscles of the upper arms, particularly the shoulders and triceps, are less muscled ("jelly roll arms"). Hands tend to be thin and wrinkly, and buttocks often sag. The inner thighs just above the knees may also sag. Bones thin, and it is not uncommon to see low growth hormone levels in people with osteoporosis. Bone loss can also thin your jaw line, and your jaw may begin to recede. With low growth hormone, your skin becomes dry and thin and there is less sweating, making you more prone to heat intolerance.

Measuring Growth Hormone

There is debate about the best way to measure growth hormone, since it is produced during our deepest sleep in the middle of the night and remains in our circulation for only a short period of time. Growth hormone is produced in response to low sugar levels and amino acids, the building blocks of protein. Classic tests used by most endocrinologists are difficult and expensive, and require infusions of amino acids such as arginine or hormones (insulin or glucagon) in your vein. For this reason, other tests are often used that may be less precise but easier to take.

Measuring IgF-1 levels indirectly measures growth hormone, because growth hormone produces its effects via a family of compounds called somatomedins, or insulin growth factors (IGFs), produced in the liver. A fasting blood test is needed for IGF-1 levels. An optimal IGF-1 level is 250 to 350 ng/ml. There is criticism that these tests are not 100 percent reliable, since this measure reflects how growth hormone affects the liver, but not necessarily our other cells. Despite its limitations, IGF-1 levels are often used to follow growth hormone injection therapy and can be used as a screening test for low growth hormone.

Twenty-four hour urine or first-morning urine tests are now available to measure growth hormone and have been used in Europe for some time. There is concern about the reliability of these urine tests, but I have found that nearly all patients who come to me with sleep problems who also test low find that the quality and depth of sleep improve after using growth hormone or growth hormone supports. So this test is a great screening test to see who is likely to respond to therapy. It can help you decide whether to invest in an expensive treatment like growth hormone injections or other growth hormone supports. Urine tests are easy to do and not too costly. On rare occasions, growth hormone deficiency will be missed by urine testing, as some people waste, or lose, growth hormone in their urine. For these people, growth hormone levels appear high in the urine, even though they may be deficient. When I have patients with the signs and symptoms of low growth hormone levels, but high or normal urinary growth hormone, I check their IGF-1 level, try GH (growth hormone) injections, or prescribe GH support to see if sleep or other symptoms improve.

If IGF-1 is low, I measure a blood prolactin level (to exclude any benign pituitary tumors). At this point I also refer patients to an endocrinologist for growth hormone stimulation tests. If IGF levels are low-normal and/or urine growth hormone is low, I generally prescribe growth hormone or a growth hormone support.

Growth Hormone Support

The building blocks of protein are called amino acids. Amino acids such as arginine, lysine, ornithine, glutamine, threonine, glycine, tryptophan, and tyrosine all stimulate growth hormone production. Unfortunately, taking these amino acids, whether by nasal spray, by mouth in food, or in supplements, will not raise your growth hormone levels, despite what advertisements might claim in your computer spam or health journals. There is only one amino acid support of which I am aware that does raise growth hormone levels and improve symptoms reliably. That is Trans-d Tropin (Trans-d).

Trans-d is an amino acid–based skin lotion, available by prescription only. It does not contain any growth hormone or other hormones, but it is made up of amino acids and fatty acids combined in such a way as to stimulate your own pituitary gland to produce growth hormone. Trans-d Tropin is expensive, but less expensive than growth hormone injections. I have found it useful to improve and deepen sleep in patients with low growth hormone levels as determined by urine testing. Because it is a pre-scription medication, its use must be monitored by a doctor. (Trans-d Tropin is available only through College Pharmacy; see chapter 7).

Using Trans-d Tropin

Trans-d is sort of a nuisance, so it is my least favorite hormone support. However, because it is so successful in restoring deep, restful sleep and improving mood and well being, I do prescribe it. It is applied in a dose of 0.5 ml to the inner forearms three times daily, five days per week. Some take their dose in drops, but using drops is difficult and not con-sistent. Using a small syringe available from the pharmacy is my pre-ferred method to measure it out. Sleep improves usually within days. Over months, as growth hormone levels normalize, the dose of Trans-d can gradually be reduced to one that is easier to manage and more affordable, about 0.3 ml twice daily. Typically, every two to three months the dose will gradually be lowered, at first to 0.4 ml three times daily, and later to 0.3 ml three times daily, and eventually to a mainte-nance dose of 0.3 ml twice daily.

When using Trans-d, usually sleep deepens in two to three days and insomnia improves within seven to ten days. As sleep improves, most people also report feeling more calm, and their problems are not so overwhelming. But using Trans-d can be a little tricky. After two to three months, you may start waking up in the middle of the night again, making you wonder if the Trans-d is still working. This is a sign that you need to drop the dose slightly (usually to 0.4 ml three times daily). This process repeats itself as your growth hormone levels slowly rise. Two to three months later, when sleep again becomes too light, the next dose reduction should be made. This is counterintuitive: as sleep lightens, the dose must be lowered. Usually, a dose adjustment is needed every two to three months. After about eight to twelve months, only a small dose is required—0.25 to 0.35 ml twice daily, in the morning and at bedtime. This is usually the lowest dose that I recommend. Below this, most people become deficient again. Some people are able to stop Trans-d altogether and maintain growth hormone levels on their own, once their insomnia is cured. If insomnia returns, however, it is usually a sign that the level has once again fallen and they have to restart the entire process. For this reason, I usually recommend staying on a constant low dose and checking your level periodically to ensure that your growth hormone is properly maintained at a normal level.

Side effects of Trans-d are mainly due to too much growth hormone stimulation. You will feel revved up or unable to fall asleep—too energized. Because growth hormone stimulates other hormones, you may need to reduce the doses of these other hormones, particularly DHEA, thyroid, estradiol, and testosterone. The increase in estradiol may cause breast tenderness or swelling. If this occurs, lower your estradiol and make sure that you are taking enough progesterone to balance your estrogen.

It is the rare patient whose symptoms and urinary growth hormone levels do not improve using Trans-d. You usually know within a week or two if it is working. Repeat your growth hormone levels to make sure your response is adequate. For some reason, IGF-1 does not always increase with Trans-d as it does with growth hormone injections. But remember, how you feel is always the best guide. If your urinary growth hormone level does not rise and/or your symptoms are no better, and you are using Trans-d three times a day, five days a week, I would try using it three times a day every day and recheck levels. If you still have no satisfactory response, then you should move on to growth hormone injections.

There are many protocols for using Trans-d, and some of these mention the need to take one- or two-week breaks from Trans-d after a month or two. I have not found this necessary. In fact, taking breaks, especially early on in treatment, can result in a return of insomnia symptoms and may lower the growth hormone level you worked so hard to establish. Some also claim that you shouldn't use Trans-d with melatonin, DHEA, or testosterone. I disagree. Trans-d will cause a rise in these hormones, as previously mentioned, and the need for these hormones will fall. Initially, I advise patients to continue to use all their hormones with the Trans-d, and monitor levels or reduce them when signs of excess arise (see appendix B).

Growth Hormone Injections

Growth hormone is available via injections only. Although effective, these shots are expensive (about $300 to 400 per month). But if you need it, and can afford it, it can turn your life around.

The recommended dose of growth hormone varies, depending upon how strong your adrenal glands are. Because growth hormone will lower your cortisol (usually by 10 to 40 percent), your starting dose will vary, depending on how well your adrenals are supported. The starting dose can be as low as 0.5 mcg per day. Over the course of several days, your dose can gradually be increased to 1.25 and then to 1.5 mcg daily. This higher dose can be reduced slowly over time when symptoms disappear. It is ideal to give injections divided into two doses, with one third of the dose in the morning, and the remaining two thirds in the evening, at bedtime. However, I find that most people prefer, and do just as well with, a single dose at bedtime. It is given subcutaneously—that is, under the skin (similar to how insulin is given). Some endocrinologists recommend using injections for one to two years, then taking a break and monitoring levels. Once sleep disorders are corrected and other hormones are supported, your body may be able to produce adequate levels on its own. Growth hormone is now available in easy-to-use, multidose dispensing pens. A very small (31G) needle is used, making the injections relatively painless. Rarely, swelling can occur due to the injection itself or from increased muscle growth. So injections into muscle should be avoided and the site of injection should be varied. Usually injections are given in the thigh or abdomen.

Side effects of too much growth hormone are dose-related and are only seen when excessive doses are used. These include swelling of the feet or hands, tingling of the fingers or nose, difficulty falling asleep, symptoms of cortisol deficiency (fatigue), or symptoms of excess sex hormones (hirsuitism, acne, oily skin, or breast tenderness—see appendix B), excessive hunger, sweating, and increased blood sugar.

Reducing the dose of growth hormone will reverse these symptoms.

Growth hormone can also cause water retention, leading to swelling of the hands or feet. This is because growth hormone can stimulate the rennin-aldosterone system. If swelling occurs, reduce the dose and take potassium aspartate (100 to 200 mg/day).

Excessive muscle development, particularly in the shoulders, can occur with excessively high doses. This is most often seen when growth hormone is abused by athletes or bodybuilders, who have normal levels of growth hormone to start with. In such instances, you may actually see signs of acromegaly, or growth hormone excess, with enlargement of the nose, chin, jaw, hands, or feet.

Growth Hormone Controversy

Growth hormone injections may be considered controversial, but they have an excellent track record for safety. Initially there were fears of increased cancer because patients who suffer from acromegaly (a disease of the pituitary gland, where excess growth hormone is produced) have an increased incidence of colon cancer. There is no evidence to support this fear. An increase in colon cancer (or any other cancer) has not been seen. To the contrary, studies have shown that patients with cancer of the gastrointestinal tract have an improved remission rate when they use growth hormone injections. Studies both large and small have failed to show any serious long-term adverse consequences from the adult use of growth hormone. The FDA has approved its use for growth hormone deficiency in adults.

At the heart of this controversy is a financial concern. Growth hormone injections are costly—a year's supply may cost upward of three to four thousand dollars. If growth hormone levels fall naturally as we age, can we afford this treatment for all aging adults? Who will decide who gets growth hormone?

If you are having problems with insomnia, weight control, bone loss, or fatigue, and other hormone treatments have not been effective, you should definitely consider growth hormone injections. If your levels are low (determined by urinary or blood tests) and you can afford it, it can improve your life and lessen aging effects long-term.

Conclusion

W ell, if I've done my job, you are now feeling encouraged, reassured, excited, curious and, I hope, not too overwhelmed by so much information. What you need to know now is how to find a caring physician who is willing to take the time to listen to your concerns and monitor your health as your body continues to change and transform. These doctors are out there, and the labs, pharmacies, and alternative medical organizations listed in chapters 6 and 7 will help you find one.

You are entitled to feel emotionally stable, energetic, and not at the mercy of your changing body and waning hormones. It is not a woman's helpless fate to suffer thorough monthly ups and downs and years of hormonal depletion. You don't need to feel bone-tired and out of control because of your oscillating hormones. You don't need to medicate and sedate yourself through menopause, and you don't need to be frightened by the latest health study warning you off hormones— the very hormones that gave you pregnancy, breast-fed your babies, and provided you with great sex and good skin. You do not need to wait for the next double-blind, statistically manipulated mega-study to tell you what is right. You know what feels right. You know that when your breasts hurt and you can't think straight, things are not right. Now you can do what you need to do to get yourself back in balance and in control of your sleep, weight, and emotions.

Remember, menopause doesn't happen overnight, and you aren't going to fix it in one day. Don't try to do everything all at once. Pick a symptom or two, decide that you are no longer going to be victimized by it, and take action.

Our Future

Womanhood is complex and amazing, and it deserves an equally amazing old age. We are, most of us, going to be living well beyond our eighties, and we are destined to spend over half of our lives on the verge of menopause, in menopause, and beyond. Most of us are going to receive twenty extra years to watch our grandchildren and great-grandchildren grow—biblical life spans, bonus years, for at least one million people.

We are the first generation of women who have the power and freedom to start second or third careers, and we won't be alone. Men are catching up with us. They are now growing old with us, and we need to be able to love them enthusiastically for a long time. We need to have bones that can make sure we play tennis and do yoga into our nineties. We need minds that will stay sharp and alert, and strong hearts that will keep us dancing. There have been some amazing medical breakthroughs in our lifetime. We baby-boomer girls have changed sex and reproduction. We have walked to raise billions of dollars to fight cancer. Breast cancer rates were coming down even before the WHI study was published. We did that, not the drug companies, and we can take women's health to the next level.

The Future of Hormones

The future of hormones is now. With a simple blood test, we can look at your DNA and determine if you are at risk for breast cancer, stroke, heart disease, dementia, or osteoporosis. Your daughter can take this same test to see if she is at risk of a stroke if she uses birth control pills. You now have the tools to learn which enzymes in your body, coded by your DNA, are sluggish, and what foods and supplements you need to move them along. You can be proactive to prevent your own heart attack and cancer. Your health doesn't have to be a crap shoot, and you don't have to succumb to your genetic shortcomings.

More and more doctors are studying healing modalities from around the world. We use acupuncture, homeopathy, meditation, yoga, prayer, herbs, massage, and physical therapy to strengthen ourselves, and we use foods medicinally to prevent and curb disease. Acupuncture will become mainstream for treating strokes. Targeted amino acid therapies will be used to treat depression, anxiety, and insomnia. Our serotonin and dopamine will be supported naturally, without medications that stifle your sex drive, drain your energy, or weaken your spirit. We will use herbs and supplements to improve our metabolism and enhance conventional treatments. In the future, our vitamins and antioxidants will be measured and monitored to make individualized vitamin supplements that will change as your environment changes.

The journey of your life as a woman should bring you the contentment, the strength, and the courage to be everything you want to be. The world needs more happy and healthy women. Be one.

Appendix A: Symptoms of Low Hormones

Symptoms of Low Estrogen

Cramps and headache with the period

Low energy *with the period*

Hot flashes and/or night sweats

Headache or worsening migraines/headaches

Constant fatigue throughout the day

Failing memory

Thinning scalp hair

Sleep that is less deep

Increased facial hair

Lower sex drive

More difficulty achieving orgasm

Moods that tend to depression, loss of joie de vivre feeling

Dry skin, dry eyes, dry vagina

Recurrent vaginitis or urinary infections

Frequent urination or increased urination during the night

Joint pains (menopausal arthritis), particularly affecting the fingers and thumbs

Wrinkles about the forehead, eyes ("crow's feet"), and mouth

Breasts that sag and are less sensitive

Bone loss on bone density testing

Increased LDL (bad cholesterol) and decreased HDL (good cholesterol)

Increased triglycerides

Symptoms of Low Progesterone

Periods that are very heavy

Menstrual cycles that are very short (that is, less than twenty-five days apart)

Midcycle bleeding or spotting

Breast that are sore, tender, and/or swollen

PMS with mood changes in the seven to fourteen days *before the menstrual cycle*

Swelling of the fingers, feet, or face *before the menstrual cycle*

Headaches *before the menstrual cycle*

Very poor sleep *before the menstrual cycle*

Swollen lower belly *before the menstrual cycle*

Loose bowels or constipation *before the menstrual cycle*

Anxiety

Irritability or restlessness

Agitated or too light sleep

Symptoms of Low Testosterone

Less confidence

Less competitiveness

Sleep that is less deep

More facial wrinkles

Lower sex drive

Constant tiredness

Muscle tone that is not what it used to be despite physical activity

Bone loss

Symptoms of Low DHEA

Less body hair and pubic hair

Less hair under the arms

Dry hair, skin, and eyes

Intolerance of loud noises

Sleep that is less deep

Sleep with fewer or no dreams

Lower sex drive

Poor memory

Frequent sickness

Bone loss on bone density test

Symptoms of Low Cortisol

Low energy, particularly as the day wears on

3 to 4 p.m. slump with desire to nap

Poor ability to handle stress, being easily angered or depressed if stressed

Digestive problems

Rashes, eczema, and/or psoriasis

Joint aches

Multiple allergies and sensitivities

Frequent sickness

Colds that linger

Sugar and/or salt cravings

Frequent heart pounding (palpitations)

Need for a lot of coffee to get through the day

Anxiety with stress

Symptoms of Low Aldosterone

Poor endurance, "running out of steam"

Frequent need to "just put my feet up for a few minutes"

Low blood pressure (systolic or top blood pressure less than 100)

Fainting or feeling faint when rising to stand, bending over, or standing too long

Frequent urination/urine is pale and abundant

Tendency to dehydrate easily

Symptoms of Low Pregnenolone

Memory loss

Joint pain

Feeling drained and having difficulty coping with stress

Colors not seeming as bright

Low blood pressure

Cravings for salty food

Symptoms of Low Thyroid

Becoming easily chilled

Cold hands and feet

Feeling very tired in the morning, difficulty getting going

Feeling better, having more energy after getting up and moving around

Having better energy when active

Stiff joints in the morning

Constipation or irregular bowel movements

Heavy periods and/or irregular periods

Tendency to put on weight easily

Thinning eyebrows or scalp hair

Dry skin

Puffy face and eyelids, particularly in the morning

Infertility

Symptoms of Low Growth Hormone

Inability to sleep deeply anymore

Difficulty getting energy back after doing too much or staying out too late

Feeling overwhelmed by problems

Anxiety without any reason

Thin and dry skin

Thinning hair

Sagging cheeks, with more pronounced lines under cheeks

Deepening skin wrinkles

Thinning upper lip

Loss of jaw line

Tendency to depression/feeling easily discouraged or isolated

Tendency to outbursts without provocation and sharp verbal retorts

Tendency to be a "drama queen"

Bone loss on bone density test

Symptoms of Low Melatonin

Looking older than you are

Difficulty falling asleep

Overactive mind when trying to fall asleep

Waking up during the night, suddenly

Not feeling rested in the morning

Feeling out of sync with the world, going to bed too late and waking up too late

Hot feet at night

Being very affected by jet lag

Difficulty falling back to sleep after waking up in the night

Depression/anxiety/memory loss

Appendix B: Symptoms of Hormone Excess

Symptoms of Excess Estrogen

Breast or nipple tenderness

Breast swelling

Vaginal spotting or heavy bleeding

Midcycle spotting (if still cycling)

Symptoms of Excess Progesterone

Periods delayed (greater than thirty-day cycle)

Depression or generally heavy feeling

Drugged or hungover feeling after oral progesterone

Symptoms of Excess Testosterone

Deeper voice

Increased body hair

If converted to estrogen

Breast or nipple tenderness

Breast swelling

Vaginal spotting or bleeding

Midcycle spotting (if still cycling)

If converted to DHT (dihydrotestosterone)

Hair loss

Acne

Increased body hair

Symptoms of Excess Cortisol

Palpitations

Hyper/anxious feeling

Insomnia, either having trouble falling asleep or waking in the night

Edema (swelling of the ankles)

Elevated blood pressure

Symptoms of Excess DHEA

Palpitations

Irritability

Insomnia

If converted to androstanedione

Hair thinning

Acne

Symptom of Excess Aldosterone

Elevated blood pressure

Symptoms of Excess Pregnenolone

Insomnia

Hyper/anxious feeling

Symptoms of Excess Thyroid Hormone

Palpitations

Hair loss

Hyper/anxious feeling

Insomnia

Afternoon fatigue (can cause lowered adrenal symptoms)

Weight loss

Diarrhea

Symptoms of Excess Melatonin

Insomnia, waking in the early hours

Vivid, unpleasant dreams (Bosch-like)

Palpitations (from excess conversion of T4 into T3)

Symptoms of Excess Growth Hormone

Edema or swelling of the limbs

Paresthesias or carpal tunnel syndrome

Hyper/anxious feeling

Insomnia

References

Introduction

Lesperance, F., Frasure-Smith, N., Koszycki, D., et al. Effects of Citalopram and Interpersonal Psychotherapy on Depression in Patients with Coronary Artery Disease. *JAMA* 2007; **297**:367–379.

1. Understanding Health and Hormones

Hertoghe, T. The "Multiple Hormone Deficiency" Theory of Aging: Is Human Senescence Mainly Caused by Multiple Hormone Deficiencies? *Ann NY Acad Sci* 2005; **1057**:448–465.

3. Hormone Safety and Metabolism

Alastair, E., Knight, M.J., Dryer, D., et al. Role of Polymorphic Human Cytochrome P450 Enzymes in Estrone Oxidation. *Cancer Epidemiology Biomarkers & Prevention* 2006; **15**:551–558.

Alexandersen, P., Tanko, L.B., Bagger, Y.Z., et al. The Long-Term Impact of 2–3 Years of Hormone Replacement Therapy on Cardiovascular Mortality and Atherosclerosis in Healthy Women. *Climacteric* 2006; **9**:108–118.

Arana, A., Varas, C., Gonzalez-Perez, A., et al. Hormone Therapy and Cerebrovascular Events: A Population-Based Nested Case-Control Study. *Menopause* 2006; **13**:730–736.

Auborn, K.J., Fan, S., Rosen, E.M., et al. Indole-3-Carbinol Is a Negative Regulator of Estrogen. *J. Nutr.* 2003; **133**:2470S–2475S.

Bagger, Y.Z., Tanko, L.B., Alexandersen, P., et al. Early Postmenopausal Hormone Therapy May Prevent Cognitive Impairment Later in Life. *Menopause* 2005; **12**:12–17.

Barrett-Connor, E., Laughlin, G.A. Hormone Therapy and Coronary Artery Calcification in Asymptomatic Postmenopausal Women: The Rancho Bernardo Study. *Menopause* 2005; **12**:40–48.

Birge, S.S. Estrogen and Stroke: A Case for Low Dose Estrogen. *Menopause: The Journal of the North American Menopause Society* 2006; **13**:719–720.

Campagnoli, C., Abba, C., Ambroggio, S., et al. Pregnancy, Progesterone and Progestins in Relation to Breast Cancer Risk. *J Steroid Biochem Mol Biol* 2005; **97**:441–450.

Canonico, Marianne, Oger, E., Plu-Bureau, G., et al. Hormone Therapy and Venous Thromboembolism among Postmenopausal Women, Impact of the Route of Estrogen Administration and Progestogens: The Esther Study. *Circulation* 2007; **115**:840–845.

Castagnetta, L., Granata, O.M., Cocciadiferro, L., et al. Sex Steroids, Carcinogenesis, and Cancer Progression. *Ann N Y Acad Sci* 2004; **1028**:233–246.

Chen, W.Y., Manson, J.E., Hankinson, S.E. Unopposed Estrogen Therapy and the Risk of Invasive Breast Cancer. *Arch Intern Med* 2006; **166**:1027–1032.

Chlebowski, R.T., Hendrix, S.L., Langer, R.D., et al. Influence of Estrogen Plus Progestin on Breast Cancer and Mammography in Healthy Postmenopausal Women: The Women's Health Initiative Randomized Trial. *JAMA* 2003; **289**:3243–3253.

Chetkowski, J.T., Meldrum, D.R., Steingold, K.A. Biologic Effects of Transdermal Estradiol. *N Engl J Med* 1986; **314**:1615–1620.

Clemons, M., Gross, P. Estrogen and the Risk of Breast Cancer. *N. Engl J Med.* 2001; **344**:276–285

Colditz, G.A. Epidemiology of Breast Cancer, Findings from the Nurses' Health Study. *Cancer* 1993; **71**:1480–1489.

Colditz, G.A., Manson, J.E., Hankinson, S.E. The Nurse's Health Study: 20 Year Conrtibution to the Understanding of Health among Women. *Journal of Women's Health* 1997; **6**:49–60.

Cribb, Alastair E. Knight, M. Joy, Dryer, Dagny, et al. Role of Polymorphic Human Cytochrome P450 Enzymes in Estrone Oxidation. *Cancer Epidemiology Biomarkers & Prevention* 2006; **15**:551–558.

Cushman, M., Kuller, L.H., Prentice, R., et al. Estrogen Plus Progestin and Risk of Venous Thrombosis. *JAMA* 2004; **292**:1573–1580.

de Lignieres, B. Effects of Progestogens on the Postmenopausal Breast. *Climacteric* 2002; **5**:229–235.

de Lignieres, B., de Vathaire, F., Fournier, S., et al. Combined Hormone Replacement Therapy and Risk of Breast Cancer in a French Cohort Study of 3175 Women. *Climacteric* 2002; **5**:332–340.

DeAssis, S., Hilakivi-Clarke, L. Timing of Dietary Estrogenic Exposures and Breast Cancer Risk. *N.Y. Acad. Sci.*, 2006; **1089**:14–35.

Dickson, R.B., Lippman, M.E. Estrogenic Regulation of Growth and Polypeptide Growth Factor Secretion in Human Breast Carcinoma. *Endocr. Rev.* 1987; **8**:29–43.

Dunkin, J., Rasgon, N., Wagner-Steh, K., et al. Reproductive Events Modify the Effects of Estrogen Replacement Therapy on Cognition in Healthy Postmenopausal Women. *Psychoneuroendocrinology* 2005; **30**:284–296.

Dunning, A.M., Healey, C.S., Pharoah, P.D., et al. A Systematic Review of Genetic Polymorphisms and Breast Cancer Risk. *Cancer Epidemiology Biomarkers & Prevention* 1999; **8**:843–844.

Fitzpatrick, L.A., Pace, C., Wiita, B. Comparison of Regimens Containing Oral Micronized Progesterone or Medroxyprogesterone Acetate on Quality of Life in Postmenopausal Woman: A Cross-Sectional Survey. *J Womens Health Gend Based Med* 2000; **9**:381–387.

Friel, P.N., Hinchcliffe, C., Wright, J.V. Hormone Replacement with Estradiol: Conventional Oral Doses Result in Excessive Exposure to Estrone. *Alternative Medicine Review*, 2005; **10**:36–41.

Gompel, et al. Antiestrogen Action of Progesterone in Breast Tissue. *Breast Cancer Res Treat* 1986; **8**:179–188.

Grodstein, F., Manson, J.E., Stampfer, M.J. Hormone Therapy and Coronary Heart Disease: The Role of Time Since Menopause and Age at Hormone Initiation. *J Womens Health* 2006; **15**:35–44.

Grodstein, F., Stampfer, M.J., Colditz, G.A., et al. Postmenopausal Hormone Use and Decreased Mortality. *N. Engl. J. Med.* 1997; **336**:1769–1775.

Grodstein, F., Stampfer, M.J., Manson, J.E., et al. Postmenopausal Estrogen and Progestin Use and the Risk of Cardiovascular Disease. *N. Engl. J. Med.* 1996; **335**:453–461.

Hall, D.C. Nutritional Influences on Estrogen Metabolism. *Applied Nutritional Science Reports.* 2001 by Advanced Nutrition Publications, Inc.

Hargove, O. An Alternative Method of Hormone Replacement Therapy Using the Natural Sex Steroids. *Infertile Repro Med Clinics North Am.* 1995; **6**:563–674.

Hulley, S.B., Grady, D. The WHI Estrogen-Alone Trial—Do Things Look Any Better? *JAMA* 2004; **291**:1769–1771.

Hulley, S., Grady, D., Bush, T., et al. Randomized Trial of Estrogen Plus Progestin for Secondary Prevention of Coronary Heart Disease in Postmenopausal Women. *JAMA* 1998; **280**:605–613.

Jensen, J., Riis, B.J., Strom, V., et al. Long-Term Effects of Percutaneous Estrogens and Oral Progesterone on Serum Lipoproteins in Postmenopausal Women. *Am J Obstet Gynecol* 1987; **156**:66–71.

Kabat, G.C., Chang, C.J., Sparano, J.A., et al. Urinary Esrogen Metabolites and Breast Cancer: A Case-control Study. *Cancer Epidemiology & Prevention* 1997; **6**:505–509.

Kon, K.K., Sakuma, I. Should Progestins Be Blamed for the Failure of Hormone Replacement Therapy to Reduce Cardiovascular Events in Randomized Controlled Trials? *Arteriosclerosis, Thrombosis, and Vascular Biology* 2004; **24**:1171–1189.

Kozakiewicz, K., Wycisk, A. Hormonal Replacement Therapy and Selective Estrogen Receptor Modulators in Prevention of Cardiovascular Disease. *Wiad Lek* 2006; **59**:377–382 (translated on Pubmed).

Kuller, L.H. Hormone Replacement Therapy and Risk of Cardiovascular Disease: Implications of the Results of the Women's Health Initiative. *Arteriscler Thromb Vasc Biol* 2003; **23**:11–16.

LeBlanc, E.S, Janowsky, J., Chan, B.K., et al. Hormone Replacement Therapy and Cognition: Systematic Review and Meta-Analysis. *JAMA* 2001; **285**:1489–1499.

Lord, R.S., Bongiovanni, B., Bralley, J.A. Estrogen Metabolism and the Diet-Cancer Connection: Rationale for Assessing the Ratio of Urinary Hydroxylated Estrogen Metabolites. *Alternative Medicine Review* 2002; **7**:112–129.

Lotinum, S., Westerlind, D.C., Turner, R.T. Tissue-Selective Effects of Continuous Release of 2 Hydroxyestrone and 16a-Hydroxyestrone on Bone, Uterus and Mammary Gland in Ovariectomized Growing Rats. *Journal of Endocrinology* 2001; **170**:165–174.

Lyytinen, H., Pukkala, E., Ylikorkala, O. Breast Cancer Risk in Postmenopausal Women Using Estrogen-Only Therapy. *Obstet Gynecol* 2006; **108**:1354–1360.

Maas, A.H., van der Graaf, Y., van der Schouw, Y.T., et al. HRT and Heart Disease: Problems and Prospects. *Maturitas* 2004; **47**:255–258.

Maas, A.H., van der Graaf, Y., van der Schouw, Y.T., et al. Rise and Fall of Hormone Therapy in Postmenopausal Women with Cardiovascular Disease. *Menopause* 2004; **11**:228–235.

Machens, K., Schmidt-Gollwitzer, K. Issues to Debate on the Women's Health Initiative (WHI) Study. Hormone Replacement Therapy: An Epidemiological Dilemma. *Human Reproduction* 2003; **18**:1992–1999.

Maki, P.M. Hormone Therapy and Cognitive Function: Is There a Critical Period for Benefit? *Neuroscience* 2006; **138**:1027–1030.

Manly, J.J., Merchant, C.A., Jacobs, D.M., et al. Endogenous Estrogen Levels and Alzheimer's Disease Among Postmenopausal Women. *American Academy of Neurology* 2000; **54**:833–843.

Manson, JoAnn E., Allison, Matthew A., Rossouw, Jacques, et al. Estrogen Therapy and Coronary-Artery Calcification. *NEJM* 2007; **356**:2591–2602.

Mendelsohn, M.E., Karas, R.H. The Time Has Come to Stop Letting the HERS Tale Wag the Dogma. *Circulation* 2001; **104**:2256–2259.

Meng, Q., Yuan, F., Goldberg, I.D. Indole-3-carbinol Is a Negative Regulator of Estrogen Receptor Signaling in Human Tumor Cells. *J.Nutr.* 2000; **130**:2927–2931.

Merz, C.N.B. Hormone Therapy and Cardiovascular Risk: Why the New Focus on Perimenopausal Women? *Adv Stud Med.* 2006; **6**:267–274.

Miller, K. Estrogen and DNA Damage: The Silent Source of Breast Cancer? *Journal of the National Cancer Institute* 2003; **95**:100–102.

Million Women Study Collaborators. Breast Cancer and Hormone-Replacement Therapy in the Million Women Study. *Lancet* 2003; **362**:419–427.

Muti, P., et al. Metabolism and Risk of Breast Cancer: A Prospective Analysis of 2:16 Hydroxyestrone Ratio in Premenopausal and Postmenopausal Women. *Cancer Epidemiology* 2000; **11**:635–640.

Muti, Paola. Estrogen Metabolism Affects Breast Cancer Risk in Premenopausal Women. *Epidemiology* 2000; **11**:635–640.

Naunton, Mark, Asmar, F., Al Hadithy, Y. Estradiol Gel: Review of the Pharmacology, Pharmacokinetics, Efficacy, and Safety in Menopausal Women. *Menopause: The Journal of the North American Menopause Society* 2006; **13**:517–527.

Nilsen, J., Brinton, R.D. Impact of Progestins on Estrogen-Induced Neuroprotection: Synergy by Progesterone and 19-Norprogesterone and Antagonism by Medroxyprogesterone Acetate. *Endocrinology* 2002; **143**:205–212.

Ottoson, U.B., Johansson, B.G., Von Schoultz, B. Subfractions of High-Density Lipoprotein Cholesterol during Estrogen Replacement Therapy: A Comparison between Progestogens and Natural Progesterone. *Am. J. Obstet Gynedol* 1987; **156**:66–71.

Pharoah, P.D., Antoniou, A., Bobrow, M., et al. Polygenic Susceptibility to Breast Cancer and Implications for Prevention. *Nat Genet* 2002; **31**:33–36.

Phillips, L.S., Langer, R.D. Postmenopausal Hormone Therapy: Critical Reappraisal and a Unified Hypothesis. *Fertil Steril* 2005; **83**:558–566.

Pisha, E., Lui, X., Constantinou, A.I., et al. Evidence That a Metabolite of Equine Estrogens, 4-Hydroxyequilenin, Induces Cellular Transformation in Vitro. *Chem Tes Toxicol* 2001; **14**(1):82–80.

Qinghui, Meng, Fang, Y., Itzhak, D., et al. Indole-3-Carbinol Is a Negative Regulator of Estrogen Receptor-A Signaling in Human Tumor Cells. *J. Nutr.* 2000; **130**:2927–2931.

Rogan, E.G. The Natural Chemopreventive Compound Indole-3-Carbinol: State of the Science. *In Vivo* 2006; **20**:221–228.

Ross, R.K., Paganini-Hill, A., Wan, P.C., et al. Effect of Hormone Replacement Therapy on Breast Cancer Risk: Estrogen versus Estrogen Plus Progestin. *J. Natl Cancer Inst* 2000; **92**:328–332.

Rossouw, J.E., Prentice, R.L., Manson, J.E. Postmenopausal Hormone Therapy and Risk of Cardiovascular Disease by Age and Years Since Menopause. *JAMA* 2007; **297**:1465–1477.

Scarabin, P-Y., Alhenc-Gelas, M., Plu-Bureau, G., et al. Effects of Oral and Transdermal Estrogen/Progesterone Regimens on Blood Coagulation and

Fibrinolysis in Postmenopausal Women: A Randomized Controlled Trial. *Arteriosclerosis, Thrombosis and Vascular Biology* 1997; **17**:3071–3078.

Scarabin, P-Y., Oger, E., Plu-Bureau, G. for the Estrogen and ThromboEmbolism Risk (ESTHER) Study Group. Differential Association of Oral and Transdermal Oestrogen-Replacement Therapy with Venous Thromboembolism Risk. *Lancet* 2003; **362**:428–432.

Schairer, C., Lubin, J., Troisi, R., et al. Menopausal Estrogen and Estrogen-Progestin Replacement Therapy and Breast Cancer Risk. *JAMA* 2000; **283**:485–491.

Seely, E.W., Walsh, B.W., Gerhard, M.D., et al. Estradiol with or without Progesterone and Ambulatory Blood Pressure in Postmenopausal Women. *Hypertension* 1999; **33**:1190–1194.

Shumaker, S.A., Legault, C., Kuller, L., et al. Conjugated Equine Estrogens and Incidence of Probable Dementia and Mild Cognitive Impairment in Postmenopausal Women. *JAMA* 2004; **291**:2947–2958.

Shumaker, S.A., Legault, C., Rapp, S.R., et al. Estrogen Plus Progestin and the Incidence of Dementia and Mild Cognitive Impairment in Postmenopausal Women. *JAMA* 2003; **289**:2651–2662.

Smith, N.L., Heckbert, S.R., Lemaitre, R., et al. Esterified Estrogens and Conjugated Equine Estrogens and the Risk of Venous Thrombosis. *JAMA* 2004; **292**:1581–1587.

Speroff, L. The Million Women Study and Breast Cancer. *Maturitas* 2003; **46**:1–6.

Stefanick, M.L., Anderson, G.L., Margolis, K.L., et al. Effects of Conjugated Equine Estrogens on Breast Cancer and Mammography Screening in Postmenopausal Women with Hysterectomy. *JAMA* 2006; **295**:1647–1667.

Tannen, Richard L., Weiner, M.G., Xie, D., et al. Estrogen Affects Post-Menopausal Women Differently Than Estrogen Plus Progestin Replacement Therapy. *Human Reproduction* 2007; **22**:1769–1777.

Thomas, T., Rhodin, J., Clark, L., et al. Progestins Initiate Adverse Events of Menopausal Estrogen Therapy. *Climacteric* 2003 **6**:293–301.

Thompsom, P.A., Ambrosne, C. Molecular Epidemiology of Genetic Polymorphisms in Estrogen Metabolizing Enzymes in Human Breast Cancer. *Journal of the National Cancer Institute Monographs* 2000; **27**:125–134.

Ursin, G., London, S., Stanczyk, F.Z. Urinary 2 Hydroxyestrone/16-Hydroxyestrone Ratio and Risk of Breast Cancer in Postmenopausal Women. *Journal of the National Cancer Institute* 1999; **91**:1067–1072.

Wassertheil-Smoller, S., Hendrix, S.L., Limacher, M., et al. Effect of Estrogen Plus Progestin on Stroke in Postmenopausal Women: The Women's Health Initiative: A Randomized Trial. *JAMA* 2003; **291**:2673–2684.

The Women's Health Initiative Steering Committee. Effects of Conjugated Equine Estrogen in Postmenopausal Women with Hysterectomy: The

Women's Health Initiative Randomized Controlled Trial. *JAMA* 2004; **291**:1701–1712.

Wright, D.W., Kellermann, A.L., Hertzberg, V.S., et al. Protect: A Randomized Clinical Trial of Progesterone for Acute Traumatic Brain Injury. *Ann Emerg Med* 2007; **49**:391–402.

Writing Group for the PEPI Study. *JAMA* 1995; **273**:199–208.

Writing Group for the Women's Health Initiative Investigators. Risks and Benefits of Estrogen Plus Progestin in Healthy Postmenopausal Women: Principal Results From the Women's Health Initiative Randomized Controlled Trial. *JAMA* 2002; **288**:321–341.

Yager, J.D. Enogenous Estrogen as Carcinogens through Metabolic Activation. *Journal of the National Cancer Institute Monographs* 2000; **27**:67–73.

Yager, J.D., Davidson, N.E. Estrogen Carcinogenesis in Breast Cancer. *N.E. Journal of Medicine* 2006; **354**:270–282.

Yang, X., Yan, L., Davidson, N.E. DNA Methylation in Breast Cancer. *Endocrine-Related Cancer* 2001; **8**:115–127.

Zandi, P.P., Carlson, M.C., Plassman, B.L., et al. Hormone Replacement Therapy and Incidence of Alzheimer Disease in Older Women: The Cache Country Study. *JAMA* 2002; **288**:2123–2129.

Zhu, B.T., Conney, A.H. Is Methoxyestradiol an Endogenous Estrogen Metabolite that Inhibits Mammary Carcinogenesis? *Cancer Research* 1998; **58**:2268–2277.

4. Hormones and a Healthy Lifestyle

Andersson, A.M., Skakkeback, N.E. Exposure to Exogenous Estrogens in Food: Possible Impact on Human Development and Health. *European Journal of Endocrinology* 1999; **140**:477–485.

Antibiotics and Breast Cancer: What's the Connection? *Emergency Medicine* 2004; November:52–54.

Awad, A.B., Roy, R., R., Fink, C.S. Beta-Sitosterol, a Plant Sterol, Induces Apoptosis and Activates Key Caspases in MDA-MB-231 Human Breast Cancer Cells. *Oncol Rep.* 2003; **10**:497–500.

Buzdar, Aman U. Dietary Modification and Risk of Breast Cancer. *JAMA* 2006; **295**:691–692.

Cornelis, M.C., El-Sohemy, A., Kabagambe, E.K., et al. Coffee, CYP1A2 Genotype, and Risk of Myocardial Infarction. *JAMA* 2006; **295**:1135–1141.

Darbre, P.D. Underarm Cosmetics and Breast Cancer. *J. App. Toxicol* 2003; **23**:89–95.

Epidemiology and Biostatistics Program, Division of Cancer Epidemiology and Genetics, National Cancer Institute, Bethesda, MD. Phytoestrogens and Breast Cancer. *American Journal of Clinical Nutrition* 2004; **79**:183–184.

Gardner, C.D., Kiazand, A., Alhassan, S., et al. Comparison of the Atkins, Zone, Ornish, and LEARN Diets for Change in Weight and Related Risk Factors among Overweight Premenopausal Women. *JAMA* 2007; **297**:969–977.

Goldstein, Larry B. Low LDL Cholesterol, Statins, and Brain Hemorrhage: Should We Worry? *Neurology* 2007; **68**:719–720.

Horn-Ross, Pamela L., Canchola, A.J., West, D.W., et al. Patterns of Alcohol Consumption and Breast Cancer Risk in the California Teachers Study Cohort. *Cancer Epidemiology Biomarkers & Prevention*, 2004; **13**:405–411.

Katan, M.B., Grundy, S.M., Jones, P., et al. Efficacy and Safety of Plant Stanols and Sterols in the Management of Blood Cholesterol Levels. *Mayo Clin Proc.* 2003; **78**:965–978.

Keinan-Boker, Lital, van Der Schouw, Y., Grobbee, D.E., et al. Dietary Phyto-estrogens and Breast Cancer Risk. *Am J Cin Nutr* 2004; **79**:282–288.

Kuriyama, S., Shimazu, T., Ohmori, K., et al. Green Tea Consumption and Mortality Due to Cardiovascular Disease, Cancer, and All Causes in Japan. *JAMA* 2006; **296**:1255–1265.

Kurzer, Mindy S. Hormonal Effects of Soy in Premenopausal Women and Men. *J. Nutr.* 2002; **132**:570S–573S.

McTiernan, A., Kooperberg, C., White, E., et al. Recreational Physical Activity and the Risk of Breast Cancer in Postmenopausal Women. *JAMA* 2003; **290**:1331–1336.

Meilahn, Elaine N. Low Serum Cholesterol Hazardous to Health? *Circulation* 1995; **92**:2365–2366.

Nanda, S., Gupta, N., Mehta, H.C., et al. Effect of Oestrogen Replacement Therapy on Serum Lipid Profile. *The Australian and New Zealand Journal of Obstetrics and Gynaecology* 2003; **43**:213–216.

Ostlund, R.E., Jr. Phytosterols in Human Nutrition. *Annu Rev Nutr.* 2002; **22**:533–549.

Perera, F.P., et al. Study Links Environmental Contaminants with Breast Cancer. *Carcinogenesis* 2000; **21**:1281–1289.

Rossouw, J.E., Prentice, R.L., Manson, J.E. Postmenopausal Hormone Therapy and Risk of Cardiovascular Disease by Age and Years since Menopause. *JAMA* 2007; **297**:1465–1477.

Singletary, K.W., Gapstur, S.M. Alcohol and Breast Cancer: Review of Epidemiologic and Experimental Evidence and Potential Mechanisms. *JAMA* 2001; **286**:2143–2151.

Smith-Warner, S.A., Spiegelman, D., Yaun, S.S., et al. Intake of Fruits and Vegetables and Risk of Breast Cancer: A Pooled Analysis of Cohort Studies. *JAMA* 2001; **285**:769–776.

Ulmer, H., Kelleher, C., Diem, G., et al. Why Eve Is Not Adam: Prospective Follow-up of 14,9650 Women and Men of Cholesterol and Other Risk Factors Related to Cardiovascular and All-Cause Mortality. *J Womens Health* 2004; **13**:41–53.

Velicer, C.M., Heckbert, S.R., Lampe, J.W. et al. Antibiotic Use in Relation to the Risk of Breast Cancer. *JAMA* 2004; **291**:827–835.

Ziegler, R.G. Phytoestrogens and Breast Cancer. *American Journal of Clinical Nutrition* 2004; **79**:183–184.

8. Sex Hormones Part 1: Perimenopause and Progesterone

Beral, V. Million Women Study Collaborators. Breast Cancer and Hormone-Replacement Therapy in the Million Women Study. *Lancet* 2003; **362**:419–427.

Brett, K.M. Can Hysterectomy Be Considered a Risk Factor for Cardiovascular Disease? *Circulation* 2005; **111**:1456–1458.

Brewster, W.R., DiSaia, P.J., Grosen, E.A., et al. HRT after Breast Cancer Part 2. *Gynecol Endocrinol* 2002; **16**:469–478.

Campagnoli, C., Abba, C., Ambroggio, S., et al. Pregnancy, Progesterone and Progestins in Relation to Breast Cancer Risk. *J Steroid Biochem Mol Biol* 2005; **97**:441–450.

Chlebowski, R.T., Hendrix, S.I., Langer, R.D., et al., for the WHI Investigators. Influence of Estrogen Plus Progestin on Breast Cancer and Mammography in Healthy Postmenopausal Women: The Women's Health Initiative Randomized Trial. *JAMA* 2003; **289**:3243–3253.

Col, N.F., Hirota, L.K., Orr, R.K., et al. Hormone Replacement Therapy after Breast Cancer: A Systematic Review and Quantitative Assessment of Risk. *F. Clin Oncol* 2001; **19**:2357–2363.

Chen, J., Chopp, M., Li, Y. Neuroprotective Effects of Progesterone after Transient Middle Cerebral Artery Occlusion in Rat. *J Neurol Sci* 1999; **171**:24–30.

Colditz. Estrogen, Estrogen Plus Progestin Therapy, and Risk of Breast Cancer. *Clin. Cancer Res.* 2005; **11**:909x–917s.

Collins, et al. Breast Cancer Risk with Postmenopausal Hormonal Treatment. *Hum Reprod Update* 2005; **11**:545–560.

Davis, et al. Postmenopausal Hormone Therapy: From Monkey Glands to Transdermal Patches. *J. Endocrinol* 2005; **185**:207–222.

de Fa, T., Sobreira, M., Clapauch, R. Comparison of Gel and Patch Estradiol Replacement in Brazil, A Tropical Country. *Maturitas* 2000; **31;36**:69–74.

de Lignieres, B. Effects of Progestogens on the Postmenopausal Breast. *Climacteric* 2002; **5**:229–235.

de Lignieres, B. Oral Micronized Progesterone. *Clin Ther* 1999; **21**:41–60.

de Lignieres, B., de Vathaire, F., Fournier, S., et al. Combined Hormone Replacement Therapy and Risk of Breast Cancer in a French Cohort Study of 3175 Women. *Climacteric* 2002; 5:332–340.

Fitzpatrick, L.A., Pace, C., Wiita, B. Comparison of Regimens Containing Oral Micronized Progesterone or Medroxyprogesterone Acetate on Quality of Life in Postmenopausal Woman: A Cross-Sectional Survey. *J Womens Health Gend Based Med* 2000; 9:381–387.

Gallagher, J. Christopher. Effect of Early Menopause on Bone Density and Fractures. *The Journal of the North American Menopause Society* 2007; 14:567–571.

Greiser, et al. Menopausal Hormone Therapy and Risk of Breast Cancer: A Meta-Analysis of Epidemiological Studies and Randomized Controlled Trials. *Human Reprod Update* 2005; 11:561–573.

Hardy, M.L. Women's Health Series: Herbs of Special Interest to Women. *J Am Pharm Assoc* 2000; 40(2):234–242.

Harman, et al. Is the Estrogen Controversy Over: Deconstructing the Women's Health Initiative Study: A Critical Evaluation of the Evidence. *Ann N.Y. Acad. Sci.* 2005; 1052:43–56.

Jeanes, Helen, L., Wanikiat, P., Sharif, I., et al. Medroxyprogesterone Acetate Inhibits the Cardioprotective Effect of Estrogen in Experimental Ischemia-Reperfusion Injury. *Menopause: The Journal of the North American Menopause Society* 2006; 13:80–86.

Jensen, J., Riis, B.J., Strom, V., et al. Long-Term Effects of Percutaneous Estrogens and Oral Progesterone on Serum Lipoproteins in Postmenopausal Women. *Am J Obstet Gynecol* 1987; 156:66–71.

Kumar, et al. Type and Duration of Exogenous Hormone Use Affects Breast Cancer Histology. *Ann. Surg. Oncol.* 2007; 14:695–703.

McPherson and Mant. Dose and Duration of Hormone Use: Understanding the Effects of Combined Menopausal Hormones on Breast Cancer Better. *Community Health* 2005; 59:1078–1079.

Naunton, M., Asmar, F., Al Hadithy, Y., et al. Estradiol Gel: Review of the Pharmacology, Pharmacokinetics, Efficacy, and Safety in Menopausal Women. *Menopause: The Journal of the North American Menopause Society* 2006; 13:517–527.

Norman, R.J., MacLennan, A.H. Current Status of Hormone Therapy and Breast Cancer. *Human Reproduction Update* 2005; 11(6): 541–543.

Ragonese, P., D'Amelio, M., Salemi, G., et al. Risk of Parkinson Disease in Women: Effect of Reproductive Characteristics. *Neurology* 2004; 62:2010–2014.

Rosano, G.M., Webb, C.M., Chierchia, S., et al. Natural Progesterone, but Not Medroxyprogesterone Acetate, Enhances the Beneficial Effect of Estrogen on Exercise-Induced Myocardial Ischemia in Postmenopausal Women. *J Am Coll Cardiol* 2000; 36:2154–2159.

Rosen, et al. BRCA1 in Hormonal Carcinogenesis: Basic and Clinical Research. *Endocr Relat Cancer* 2005; **12**:533–548.

Ryan, N, Rosner, A. Qualtiy of Life and Costs Associated with Micronized Progesterone and Medroxyprogesterone in Hormone Replacement Therapy for Non-hysterectomized, Postmenopausal Women. *Clin Ther* 2001; **23**:1099–1115.

Scarabin, P-Y., Alhenc-Gelas, M., Plu-Bureau, G., et al. Effects of Oral and Transdermal Estrogen/Progesterone Regimens on Blood Coagulation and Fibrinolysis in Postmenopausal Women: A Randomized Controlled Trial. *Arteriosclerosis, Thrombosis and Vascular Biology* 1997; **17**:3071–3078.

Scarabin, P-Y., Oger, E., Plu-Bureau, G., for the Estrogen and ThromboEmbolism Risk (ESTHER) Study Group. Differential Association of Oral and Transdermal Oestrogen-Replacement Therapy with Venous Thromboembolism Risk. *Lancet* 2003; **362**:428–432.

Schairer, Catherine, Lubin, J, Troisi, R, et al. Menopausal Estrogen and Estrogen-Progestin Replacement Therapy and Breast Cancer Risk. *JAMA* 2000; **283**:485–491.

Schumacher, Michael, Guennoun, R, Ghoumari, A, et al. Novel Perspectives for Progesterone in Hormone Replacement Therapy, with Special Reference to the Nervous System. *Endocrine Reviews* 2007; **28**:387–439.

Shantakumar, et al. Age and Menopausal Effects of Hormonal Birth Control and Hormone Replacement Therapy in Relation to Breast Cancer Risk. *Am J Epidemiol* 2007; **165**:1187–1198.

Stefanick, et al. Effects of Conjugated Equine Estrogens on Breast Cancer and Mammography Screening in Postmenopausal Women with Hysterectomy. *JAMA* 2006; **295**:1647–1657.

Thomas, T., Rhodin, J., Clark, L., et al. Progestins Initiate Adverse Events of Menopausal Estrogen Therapy. *Climacteric* 2003; **6**:293–301.

Vehkavaara, S., Silveira, A., Hakala-Ala-Pietile, T., et al. Effects of Oral and Transdermal Estrogen Replacement Therapy on Markers of Coagulation, Fibrinolysis, Inflammation and Serum Lipids and Lipoproteins in Postmenopausal Women. *Thromb Haemost* 2001; **85**:619–625.

Wepfer, S.T. The Science behind Bioidentical Hormone Replacement Therapy. *International Journal of Pharmaceutical Compounding* 2001; **5**:10–12.

Wood, Charles E., Sitruk-Ware, R L., Tsong,Y, et al. Effects of Estradiol with Oral or Intravaginal Progesterone on Risk Markers for Breast Cancer in a Postmenopausal Money Model. *Menopause: The Journal of North American Menopause Society* 2007; **14**:639–647.

Wright, D.W., Kellermann, A.L., Hertzberg, V.S., et al. Protect: A Randomized Clinical Trial of Progesterone for Acute Traumatic Brain Injury. *Ann Emerg Med* 2007; **49**:391–402.

Yager and Davidson. Estrogen Carcinogenesis in Breast Cancer. *NEJM* 2006; **354**:270–282.

9. Sex Hormones Part 2: Using Natural Bioidentical Estrogen and Testosterone

Alexandersen, P., Tanko, L.B., Bagger, Y.Z., et al. The Long-Term Impact of 2–3 Years of Hormone Replacement Therapy on Cardiovascular Mortality and Atherosclerosis in Healthy Women. *Climacteric* 2006; **9**:108–118.

Alonso de Lecinana, M., Egido, J.A., Fernandez, C., et al. Risk of Ischemic Stroke and Lifetime Estrogen Exposure. *Neurology* 2007; **68**:33–38.

Antoine, C., Liebens, F., Carly, B., et al. Safety of Hormone Therapy after Breast Cancer: A Qualitative Systematic Review. *Human Reproduction* 2007; **22**:616–622.

Archer, Johanna, Love-Geffen, T E., Herbst-Damm, Kathryn L., et al. Effect of Estradiol versus Estradiol and Testosterone on Brain-Activation Patterns in Postmenopausal Women. *Menopause* 2006; **13**:528–537.

Bagger, Y.Z., Tanko, L B., Alexandersen, P, et al. Early Postmenopausal Hormone Therapy May Prevent Cognitive Impairment Later in Life. *Menopause* 2005; **12**:12–17.

Barlow, et al. Prospective Breast Cancer Risk Prediction Model for Women Undergoing Screening Mammography. *JNCI J Natl Cancer Inst* 2006; **98**:1204–1214.

Barrett-Connor, E., Laughlin, G.A. Hormone Therapy and Coronary Artery Calcification in Asymptomatic Postmenopausal Women: The Rancho Bernardo Study. *Menopause* 2005; **12**:40–48.

Baton, Matthias, Meyer, Matthias, Haas, Elvira. Hormone Replacement Therapy and Atherosclerosis in Postmenopausal Women: Does Aging Limit Therapeutic Benefits? *Arterioscler Thromb Vasc Biol.* 2007; **27**: 1669–1672.

Boccardi, Marina, Ghidoni, R., Govoni, S., et al. Effects of Hormone Therapy on Brain Morphology of Healthy Postmenopausal Women: A Voxel-Based Morphometry Study. *Menopause* 2006; **13**:584–591.

Brett, K.M. Can Hysterectomy Be Considered a Risk Factor for Cardiovascular Disease? *Circulation* 2005; **111**:1456–1458.

Brubaker. Effects of Estrogen-Only Treatment in Postmenopausal Women. *JAMA* 2004; **292**:686–686.

Bush, Trudy, L., Whiteman, M, Flaws, J, A. *Hormone Replacement Therapy and Breast Cancer: A Qualitative Review* 2001; **98**:498–508.

Canonico, Marianne, Oger, E., Plu-Bureau, G., et al. Hormone Therapy and Venous Thromboembolism Among Postmenopausal Women, Impact of the Route of Estrogen Administration and Progestogens: The Esther Study. *Circulation* 2007; **115**:840–845.

Chen, W.Y., Manson, J.E., Hankinson, S.E. Unopposed Estrogen Therapy and the Risk of Invasive Breast Cancer. *Arch Intern Med* 2006; **166**:1027–1032.

Chetkowski, R.J., Meldrum, D.R., Steingold, K.A., et al. Biologic Effects of Transdermal Estradiol. *N.E. Journal of Medicine* 1986; **314**:1615–1620.

Cimicifuga Racemosa. *Alternative Medicine Review* 2003; **8**:186–192.

Collins, Peter, Guiseppe, G., Casey, C., et al. Management of Cardiovascular Risk in the Peri-Menopausal Woman: A Consensus Statement of European Cardiologists and Gynaecologists. *European Heart Journal* 2007 (advance publication).

Coombs, et al. Hormone Replacement Therapy and Breast Cancer: Estimate of Risk. *BMJ* 2005; **331**:347–349.

de Lecinana, M. Alonso, Egido, J.A, Fernandez, C., et al. Risk of Ischemic Stroke and Lifetime Estrogen Exposure. *Neurology* 2007; **68**:33–38.

Dunkin, J., Rasgon, N., Wagner-Steh, K., et al. Reproductive Events Modify the Effects of Estrogen Replacement Therapy on Cognition in Healthy Post-menopausal Women. *Psychoneuroendocrinology* 2005; **30**:284–296.

Durna, E.M., Wren, B.G., Heller, G.Z., et al. *Hormone Replacement Therapy After a Diagnosis of Breast Cancer: Cancer Recurrence and Mortality*, MJA 2002; **177**(7):347–351.

Fournier, A., Berrino, F., Riboli, E., et al. Breast Cancer Risk in Relation to Different Types of Hormone Replacement Therapy in the E3N-EPIC Cohort. *Int J Cancer* 2005; **114**:448–454.

Gallagher, J. Christopher. Effect of Early Menopause on Bone Density and Fractures. *The Journal of the North American Menopause Society* 2007; **14**:567–571.

Goldberg, C. Removal of Ovaries May Affect Heart. *Boston Globe—Source: Obstetrics & Gynecology*, Aug. 1, 2005.

Goldstein, Larry B. Low LDL Cholesterol, Statins, and Brain Hemorrhage: Should We Worry? *Neurology* 2007; **68**:719–720.

Gonnelli, S., Cepollaro, C., Pondrelli, C., et al. The Usefulness of Bone Turnover in Predicting the Response to Transdermal Estrogen Therapy in Postmenopausal Osteoporosis. *Journal of Bone and Mineral Research* 1997; **12**:624–631.

Grodstein, F., Manson, J.E., Stampfer, M.J. Hormone Therapy and Coronary Heart Disease: The Role of Time since Menopause and Age at Hormone Initiation. *J Womens Health* 2006; **15**:35–44.

Henderson, Victor W., Sherwin, B.B. Surgical Versus Natural Menopause: Cognitive Issues. *Menopause* 2007; **14**:572–579.

Hirschberg, Angelica L., Edlund, Mans, Svane, Gunilla, et al. An Isopropanolic Extract of Black Cohosh Does Not Increase Mammographic Breast Density or Breast Cell Proliferation in Postmenopausal Women. *Menopause: The Journal of the North American Menopause Society* 2007; **14**:89–96.

Howard, B.V., Kuller, L., Langer, R., et al. Risk of Cardiovascular Disease by Hysterectomy Status, with and without Oophorectomy. The Women's Health Initiative Observational Study. *Circulation* 2005; **111**:1462–1470.

Hsia, J., Langer, R.D., Manson, J.E., et al. Conjugated Equine Estrogens and Coronary Heart Disease. *The Women's Health Initiative Arch Intern Med* 2006; **166**:357–365.

Jensen, J., Riis, B.J., Strom, V., et al. Long-Term Effects of Percutaneous Estrogens and Oral Progesterone on Serum Lipoproteins in Postmenopausal Women. *Am J Obstet Gynecol* 1987; **156**:66–71.

Joffe, Hadine, Hall, J., Gruber, S., et al. Estrogen Therapy Selectively Enhances Prefrontal Cognitive Processes: A Randomized, Double-Blind, Placebo-Controlled Study With Functional Magnetic Resonance Imaging in Perimenopausal and Recently Postmenopausal Women. *Menopause* 2006; **13**:411–422.

Kligler, B. Black Cohosh. *American Family Physician* 2003; **68**(1):114–116.

Leiblum, Sandra R., Koochaki, P.E., Rodenberg, C.A., et al. Hypoactive Sexual Desire Disorder in Postmenopausal Women: US Results from the Women's International Study of Health and Sexuality (WISHES). *Menopause* 2006; **13**:46–56.

Lemon, H.M., Wotiz H.H., Parsons, L., et al. Reduced Estriol Excretion in Patients with Breast Cancer Prior to Endocrine Therapy. *JAMA* 1966; **196**:1128–1136.

Lobo, Rogerio. Surgical Menopause and Cardiovascular Risks. *Menopause* 2007; **14**:562–566.

Maas, A.H., van der Graaf, Y., van der Schouw, Y.T., et al. HRT and Heart Disease: Problems and Prospects. *Maturitas* 2004; **47**:255–258.

Maas, A.H., van der Graaf, Y., van der Schouw, Y.T., et al. Rise and Fall of Hormone Therapy in Postmenopausal Women with Cardiovascular Disease. *Menopause* 2004; **11**:228–235.

MacLennan, Alastair H., Henderson, V.W., Paine, B.J., et al. Hormone Therapy, Timing of Initiation, and Cognition in Women Aged Older Than 60 years: The Remember Pilot Study. *Menopause* 2006; **13**:28–36.

Maki, P.M. Hormone Therapy and Cognitive Function: Is There a Critical Period for Benefit? *Neuroscience* 2006; **138**:1027–1030.

Manson, JoAnn E., Allison, Matthew A., Rossouw, Jacques, et al. Estrogen Therapy and Coronary-Artery Calcification. *NEJM* 2007; **356**:2591–2602.

Manson, JoAnn E., Bassuk, Shari, S. Invited Commentary: Hormone Therapy and Risk of Coronary Heart Disease—Why Renew the Focus on the Early Years of Menopause? *American Journal of Epidemiology* 2007; **166**:511–517.

Naessen, Tord, Lindmark, B., Lagerstrom, C., et al. Early Postmenopausal Hormone Therapy Improves Postural Balance. *Menopause* 2007; **14**:14–19.

Nanda, S., Gupta, N., Mehta, H.C., et al. Effect of Oestrogen Replacement Therapy on Serum Lipid Profile. *The Australian and New Zealand Journal of Obstetrics and Gynaecology* 2003; **43**:213–216.

Naunton, Mark, Al Hadithy, Asmar F.Y. Estradiol Gel: Review of the Pharmacology, Pharmacokinetics, Efficacy, and Safety in Menopausal Women. *Menopause: The Journal of the North American Menopause Society* 2006; **13**:517–527.

Paganini-Hill, Annlia, Corrada, Maria M., Kawas, Claudia, H. Increased Longevity in Older Users of Postmenopausal Estrogen Therapy: The Leisure World Cohort Study. *Menopause* 2006; **13**:12–18.

Parker, W.H., et al. Ovarian Conservation at the Time of Hysterectomy for Benign Disease. *Obstet Gynecol* 2005; **106**:219–226.

Peters, G.N., Fodera, T., Sabol, J., et al. Estrogen Replacement Therapy after Breast Cancer: A 12-Year Follow-Up. *Annals of Surgical Oncology* 2001; **8**(10):828–832.

Prokai-Tatrai and Prokai. Impact of Metabolism on the Safety of Estrogen Therapy. *Ann. N.Y. Acad. Sci.* 2005; **1052**:243–257.

Raus, Karel, Brucker, C, Gorkow, C, et al. First-Time Proof of Endometrial Safety of the Special Black Cohosh Extract. *Menopause* 2006; **13**:678–691.

Ravdin, Peter M., Cronin, K, A., Howlader, N, et al. The Decrease in Breast-Cancer Incidence in 2003 in the United States. *N Engl J of Med* 2007; **356**:1670–1674.

Raz, R, Stamm, W.E. A Controlled Trial of Intravaginal Estriol in Postmenopausal Women with Recurrent Urinary Tract Infections. *N Engl J Med.* 1991; **329**:753–756.

Rossouw, J.E., Prentice, R.L., Manson, J.E. Postmenopausal Hormone Therapy and Risk of Cardiovascular Disease by Age and Years since Menopause. *JAMA* 2007; **297**:1465–1477.

Scarabin, P-Y., Oger, E., Plu-Bureau. Differential Association of Oral and Transdermal Oestrogen-Replacement Therapy with Venous Thromboembolism Risk. *Lancet* 2003; **362**:428–432.

Smith, N.L., Heckbert, S.R., Lemaitre, R., et al. Esterified Estrogens and Conjugated Equine Estrogens and the Risk of Venous Thrombosis. *JAMA* 2004; **292**:1581–1587.

Tannen, Richard L., Weiner, M G., Xie, D, et al. Estrogen Affects Post-Menopausal Women Differently Than Estrogen Plus Progestin Replacement Therapy. *Human Reproduction* 2007; **22**:1769–1777.

Taylor, Hugh S. Fewer Wrinkles and Firmer Skin Linked to Earlier Use of Estrogen Therapy. *Fertility and Sterility* 2005; **84**:285–288.

Travassos de F.A., Melia Sobreira, G.M., Clapauch, R. Comparison of Gel and Patch Estraiol Replacement in Brazil, a Tropical Country. *Maturitas* **36**:69–74.

Vehkavaara, S., Silveira, A., Hakala-Ala-Pietile, T., et al. Effects of Oral and Transdermal Estrogen Replacement Therapy on Markers of Coagulation, Fibrinolysis, Inflammation and Serum Lipids and Lipoproteins in Post-menopausal Women. *Thromb Haemost* 2001; **85**:619–625.

Warnock, J.K., Swanson, S.G., Borel, R.W., et al. Combined Esterified Estrogens and Methyltestosterone Versus Esterified Estrogens Alone in the Treatment of Loss of Sexual Interest in Surgically Menopausal Women. *Menopause* 2005; **12**:374–384.

Yager, J.D., Davidson, N.E. Estrogen Carcinogenesis in Breast Cancer. *New Engl J Med* 2006; **354**:270–282.

Zandi, P.P, Carlson, M.C., Plassman, B.L., et al. Hormone Replacement Therapy and Incidence of Alzheimer Disease in Older Women: The Cache County Study. *JAMA* 2002; **288**:2123–2129.

Zhu, B.T., Conney, A.H. Is Methoxyestradiol an Endogenous Estrogen Metabolite that Inhibits Mammary Carcinogenesis? *Cancer Research* 1998; **58**:2268–2277.

10. Adrenal and Thyroid Hormones

Frey, Felix, Ferrari, P. Pastis and Hypertension—What Is the Molecular Basis. *Nephrol Dial Transplant* 2000; **15**:1512–1514.

Gaby, A.R. "Sub-Laboratory" Hypothyroidism and the Empirical Use of Armour Thyroid. *Altern Med Rev* 2004; **9**:157–179.

Ghent, W.R., Eskin, B.A., Low, D.A., et al. Iodine Replacement in Fibrocystic Disease of the Breast. *Canadian Journal of Surgery* 1993; **36**:453–460.

Hackbert, L., Heiman, J.R. Acute Dehydroepiandrosterone (DHEA) Effects on Sexual Arousal in Postmenopausal Women. *J Womens Health Gend Based Med* 2002; **11**:155–162.

Joffe, R.T., Marriott, M. Thyroid Hormone Levels and Recurrence of Major Depression. *Am J. Psychiatry* 2000; **157**:1689–1691.

Labrie, F., Belanger, A., Cusan, L., et al. Marked Decline in Serum Concentrations of Adrenal C19 Sex Steroid Precursors and Conjugated Androgen Metabolites during Aging. *J. Clin Endocrinol Metab.* 1997; **82**:2396–2402.

Oelkers, W. Dehydroepiandrosterone for Adrenal Insufficiency. *N Engl J Med.* 1999; **341**:1073–1074.

Sun, Y., Mao, M. Sun, L., et al. Treatment of Osteoporosis in Men Using Dehydroepiandrosterone Sulfate. *Chin Med. J. (Engl)* 2002; **115**:402–404.

Vallee, M., Mayo, W., LeMoal, M. Role of Pregnenolone, Dehydroepiandrosterone and Their Sulfate Esters on Learning and Memory in Cognitive Aging. *Brain Res Rev* 2001; **37**:301–312.

Villareal, D.T., Holloszy, J.O. Effect of DHEA on Abdominal Fat and Insulin Action in Elderly Women and Men: A Randomized Controlled Trial. *JAMA* 2004; **292**:2243–2248.

Wiebke, A., Callies, F., Van Vlijmen, J.C. Dehydroepiandrosterone Replacement in Women With Adrenal Insufficiency. *N Engl J Med.* 1999; **341**: 1013–1020.

11. Sleep Hormones

Arendt, J. Melatonin, Circadian Rhythms, and Sleep. *MEJM* 2000; **343**: 1115–1116.

Hertoghe, T.M., Hertoghe, T.H., Gadomski, A., et al. Melatonin and Sleep: A Review. *J Eur Anti-Aging Med.* 2005; **1**:32–37.

Sherman, B., Wysham, C., Pfohl, B. Age-Related Changes in the Circadian Rhythm of Plasma Cortisol in Man. *J.Clin Endocrinol Metab.* 1985; **61**:439–443.

Vgontzas, A.N., Zoumakis, M., Bixler, E.O., et al. Impaired Night-Time Sleep in Healthy Old versus Young Adults in Associated with Elevated Plasma Interleukin-6 and Cortisol Levels: Physiologic and Therapeutic Implications. *J. Clin Endocrinol Metab.* 2003; **88**:2087–2095.

12. Growth Hormones

Blackman, M.R., Sorkin, J.D., Munzer, T., et al. Growth Hormone and Sex Steroid Administration in Healthy Aged Men and Women, a Randomized Trial. *JAMA*, 2003; **288**:2282–2292.

Braverman, E.R. Use of Growth Hormone in Elderly Individuals. *JAMA* 2003; **290**:4.

Brooke, A.M., Monson, J.P. Adult Growth Hormone Deficiency. *Clin Med* 2003; **3**:15–19.

Gotherstrom, G., et al. A Prospective Study of 5 Years of GH Replacement Therapy in GH-Deficient Adults: Sustained Effects on Body Composition, Bone Mass, and Metabolic Indices. *Journal of Clinical Endocrinology and Metabolism*, 2001; **86**:4657–4665.

Suggested Readings

Brownstein, David, M.D. *Overcoming Thyroid Disorders*. West Bloomfield, MI: Medical Alternatives Press, 2002.

Gaby, Alan, M.D. *Preventing and Reversing Osteoporosis*. Rocklin, CA: Prima Publishing, 1994.

Hertoghe, Thierry. *The Hormone Solution*. New York: Harmony Books, 2002.

Jeffries, William M.D. *Safe Uses of Cortisol*. Springfield, IL: Charles C Thomas, 1996.

Wilson, C.A. *Adrenal Fatigue: The 21st-Century Stress Syndrome*. Petaluma, CA: Smart Publications, 2001.

Zhao, Xiaolan. *Ancient Healing for Modern Women*. New York: Walker and Company, 2006.

Index

ACTH, 197
acupuncture, 2–3, 129
Addison's disease, 197
adrenal hormones, 177–178
  adrenal glands, 7, 9
  cascade, 191
  case examples, 213–218
  common problems involving, 178–179
  hypoadrenia and, 180–182
  for jet lag, 230
  low adrenal/low thyroid symptoms,
    180–190, 247–248
  measuring, 23–24, 104, 196–198
  mood and, 93–95
  normal adrenal function, 190–198
  progesterone and, 130
  sources of extracts, 206
  supporting, with bioidentical
    hormones, 25, 199–206
  supporting, with herbs and vitamins,
    207–208
  thyroid and, 179–180, 208–213
  See also aldosterone; cortisol; DHEA
    (dehydroepiandrosterone);
    epinephrine (EPI); pregnenolone;
    thyroid hormones
adrenaline. *See* epinephrine (EPI)
aging, 2, 7, 14–16, 27, 242
  growth hormone and, 233–240

hormone support after sixty, 157
  of ovaries, 137–138
  premature, 95–97
  sleep problems and, 222
ALCAT Worldwide, 105
alcohol, 77, 226
aldosterone, 195
  fatigue and, 92
  high, 252
  low, 247–248
  measuring, 198
  mood and, 95
  supporting, 205
  See also adrenal hormones
Allopregnanolone, 121
American Academy of Anti-Aging
    Medicine, 113
American Association of Naturopathic
    Physicians, 113
American College for Advancement in
    Medicine, 113
American Holistic Medical Association,
    114
American Journal of Cardiology, 62
*American Journal of Obstetrics and
    Gynecology*, 161
amino acids, 26
  growth hormone and, 236–237
  therapies, 165

andropause, 15
androstanedione, 203–204, 252
antibodies, thyroid, 185–186, 190
antidepressants, 93–95, 143–144. *See also*
    prescription drugs
antioxidants, 42, 49, 73–77
appearance, aging and, 95–97
Armour thyroid, 209, 210
ashwagandha, 207
astragalus, 207
Ayurvedic medicine, 2

beta-sitosterol, 72–73, 129
Biestrogen, 149
bioidentical hormones, 5, 17
    estrogen, 148
    myths and facts about, 37–39
    See also hormone support therapy
        (HST); *individual types of hormones*
biotin, 171–172
Bird's Hill Pharmacy, 112
birth control
    hormone support and, 159
    pills, 6–7
bisphenol-A, 79
black cohosh, 165
bladderwrack, 212–213
blood clotting, 147–148, 157
blood tests, 102–103. *See also* lab testing
body temperature, sleep and, 226
bone fractures/loss, 35, 146, 161
bound hormones, 100–101
bovine extract, 206
bowels, 51–53
BRCA genes, 54
breakdown, of hormones. *See* hormone
    metabolism
breast cancer, 36–37
    bioidentical hormones for, 5
    diet and, 66–67
    estrogen and, 148, 164
    genetic testing and, 53–55
    glucuronidation, 50
    hormone use after, 167
    methylation, 50–51
    progesterone for, 37
    See also cancer

breast tenderness, 73, 128–130, 153, 173,
    188, 238–239
B vitamins, 129
    in methylation, 42

caffeine, 75–76, 226
calcium-d-glucarate, 53
cancer
    bioidentical hormones for, 5
    bowels and digestion, 51–53
    diet and, 66–67
    estrogen and, 148
    fear of hormones and, 18–20
    genetic testing and, 53–55
    See also breast cancer
carcinogens, 31, 78–79. *See also* breast
    cancer; cancer
CBC (complete blood count) test,
    104
chasteberry, 128
chemistry panel blood test, 104
chewing, 52
Chinese medicine, 3
    herbal blends, 129, 165, 173
    kidney yin deficiency (low adrenal),
        8–9, 83–84, 179
    kidney yang deficiency (low thyroid),
        179
    liver according to, 43–51
    perspective on symptoms, 83–84
cholesterol, 61–63
circadian rhythms, 224
Clavey, Steven, 4
Clinical Journal of Nutrition, 71
clitoral testosterone, 174
coffee, 75–76, 226
College Pharmacy, 112
compounded hormones, 38–39
    cortisol 200–201
    DHEA 203–204
    estrogen as lotions, 149–150
    progesterone 122–124
    testosterone, 173–174
    thyroid 208–210
compounding pharmacies
    finding, 111–113
    partnering with, 22–23

conjugation, 50
CoQ10, 74
cordyceps, 207–208
Cortef, 200–202
cortisol, 9, 179, 192–193
  bioidentical, 200–202
  cortisol curves, 193
  dose, 200–202
  fatigue and, 92
  high, 252
  low, 185, 247
  measuring, 196–197
  mood and, 95
  premature aging and, 97
  sex drive and, 98
  sleep and, 90–91
  See also adrenal hormones
coumestans, 72
Crinone gel, 127
cruciferous vegetables, 67–69

decaffeinated coffee, 76
dementia, 157
depression, sleep and, 223
DHEA (dehydroepiandrosterone), 7–10,
    185, 194
  DHEA-S level, 190, 197–198
  dose, 203–204
  fatigue and, 92
  high, 252
  low, 185
  measuring, 190, 197–198
  mood and, 93–95
  premature aging and, 97
  sex drive and, 98
  sleep and, 89, 91
  usage, 202–204
  See also adrenal hormones
DHT (dihydrotestosterone), 170–171, 252
diet, 26, 59–60
  antioxidants in, 49–50
  breast cancer and, 66–67
  caffeine in, 75–76, 226
  cancer and, 66
  cholesterol and, 61–63
  estrogen metabolism and, 67–78
  fats in, 60–66
  hormones from foods, 31

lemon water in, 47
  melatonin and, 225
  progesterone and, 132
  thyroid function and, 211–213
dietary fats
  cholesterol and, 61–63
  heart disease and, 60–61
  need for, 64–66
  problems of, 63–64
  See also diet
digestion, 51–53
diindolylmethane (DIM), 68
doctors
  finding, 109–110, 113–114
  "naturalist," 1
  partnering with, 22–23
Doctor's Data, Inc., 105
dong quai, 130
dopamine, 93
dosage
  cortisol, 201
  DHEA, 202–204
  estrogen, 152–156
  Florinef, 205
  growth hormone support, 237–240
  melatonin, 227–229
  pregnenolone, 204
  progesterone, 123–124
  thyroid medication, 210
  See also individual names of hormones
duration, of hormone support, 156–158

"early bird" behavior, 224
EGCG (epigallocatechin gallate), 75
Endocrine Review, 121
energy flow, liver and, 43
energy level, 84, 91–93. *See also individual
    names of hormones*
environmental pollutants, 78–79, 185
enzymes, 48, 52
epinephrine (EPI), 179, 195–196
  measuring, 198
  supporting, 206
  See also adrenal hormones
erectile dysfunction, 98
erythropoietin, 7
essential fatty acids, 64–66, 129–130
ESTHER study, 157

estradiol (E2), 40, 139, 140–141
    in compounded lotions, 149
    fatigue and, 92
    low, 142, 143–144
    measuring, 103, 104
    melatonin and, 223
    non-lotion forms of, 150
    vaginal preparations, 151–160
    See also estrogen
estriol (E3), 140, 141
    in compounded lotions, 149
    vaginal preparations, 151–160
    See also estrogen
estrogen, 24–25
    after breast cancer, 167
    after hysterectomy, 163
    bioidentical products, 148
    breast cancer and, 164
    case examples, 157–160, 161–163
    cycling of, 142–143
    defined, 138–140
    foods and metabolism of, 67–78
    genetics and, 53–54
    herbs and vitamin support for,
        164–167
    high, 251
    hysterectomy and, 160–163
    low, 143–145, 245–246
    measuring, 103, 104
    metabolism of, 40–43
    mood and, 95
    ovarian decline and, 137–138
    premature aging and, 96, 97
    preparations, 149–150, 151–160
    safe use of, 54–55, 147–148
    sleep and, 89, 91
    testosterone and, 168–175,
        251–252
    timing of, 35–37
    transitioning into menopause and,
        145–146
    types of, 140–141
    unbalanced, 117–118
    See also progesterone
estrone (E1), 40–43, 139, 140
    See also estrogen
evening primrose oil, 165
exercise, 77–78

fatigue, 92–93, 143, 178–179, 200–201,
    234
FDA (Food and Drug Administration),
    38–39
compounding pharmacies and, 111
fear, about hormones, 17–20, 241–243.
        See also safety
female pattern hair loss, 172
ferritin, 190
fibrocystic breast disease, 73, 161–162,
    188
flax
    lignans in, 70–71
    meal (ground), 53
Florinef, 205
food. See diet
4-hydoxyestrone (4-OH estrone), 42
free hormones, 100–101
free radicals
    antioxidants and, 49
    quinones, 42
fruits, antioxidants in, 73–74. See also diet
functional low thyroid, 183–185

GABA (gamma-aminobutyric acid), 93
gels
    estrogen, 154
    testosterone, 174
genetics testing, 53–55, 242–243
Genova Diagnostics, 106
Gibb, Gerald, 2–3
gingko, 207
ginseng, 207
glucuronidase, 51–52
glucuronidation, 50
goitrogens, 211
Great Plains Laboratory, Inc., 106
green tea, 75–76
growth hormone, 25, 233–234
    anxiety and, 234
    controvery about, 240
    cost, 239
    fatigue and, 93
    high, 253
    low, 234–235, 248–249
    measuring, 235–236
    mood and, 94, 95
    premature aging and, 96–97, 97

sex drive and, 98
sleep and, 91
support, 236–240

hair loss, 171–173
HDL, 61–63,121
health maintenance, 27, 146
heart disease, 32, 58–59, 156–157
    cholesterol and, 61–63
    duration of hormone support and,
        156–158
    fats and, 60–61
    recommendations to reduce, 65–66
    See also diet
Heart/Progestin Replacement Study
    (HERS), 33, 35
herbs, 26, 53
    for adrenal hormones, 207–208
    for menopausal symptoms, 164–167
    for progesterone, 127–131
    Shou Wu Wan, 173
    for thyroid, 207–208, 211–213
Hertoghe, Theirry, 8
Hippocrates, 59
homocysteine, 51, 55, 104
hormone metabolism, 40–43
    bowels and, 51–53
    estrogen, safe use of, 54–55
    estrogen and genetics, 53–54
    liver and, 43–51
    monitoring, 26
    qi and, 45–46
    See also lab testing; safety
hormone replacement therapy (HRT), 17
hormones
    balance of, 11–12
    bioidentical, explained, 5, 17, 37–39,
        148
    in meat, dairy, 66–67
    ten-step makeover, 21–27
    testing risk factors and, 53–55,
        242–243
    understanding, 13–20
    See also hormone metabolism;
        hormone support therapy (HST);
        lab testing; symptoms; *individual
        names of hormones*
hormone support therapy (HST)
    after breast cancer, 167

after hysterectomy, 160–163
defined, 17
tapering off/adjusting, 26–27
timing of, 35–37
See also individual names of hormones
horse hormones, 4–5, 206
    Premarin, 7–8, 33–35, 118
    studies involving, 30–31
hydrocortisone, 200–202
hypoadrenia (low adrenal function),
    180–182
hypothalamus, 182
hysterectomy, 160–163
    bone loss and, 161
    heart disease and, 161

Igenex Labs, 106
IgF-1 levels, 235–236
Indian ginseng, 207
indole-3-carbinol (I3C), 41–42, 67–69
injections
    for growth hormone, 239–240
    of progesterone, 127
Institute for Functional Medicine, 114
insulin growth factors, 235–236
International Academy of Compounding
        Pharmacists (IACP), 22–23, 111,
        112
iodine deficiency, 183, 186–188
iron
    deficiency, 185
    testing levels of, 190
isoflavones, 69–70

kidneys, 7
Korean ginseng, 207

lab testing, 99–100
    for adrenal hormones, 196–198
    baseline testing, 23–24
    blood tests, 102–103
    digestion and, 52
    free/bound hormones and, 100–101
    genetic, 53–55, 242–243
    growth hormone, 235–236
    for hair-loss treatment, 172
    for melatonin, 224–225
    menopause and, 146
    during menstruation, 103, 104

saliva tests, 102, 103, 105
sex hormone binding globulin
    (SHBG) and, 101
specialty labs for, 105–107
for thyroid, 23–24, 103, 188–190
timing of, 102
urine tests, 46, 102, 104–105, 189–190,
    196–197, 198, 236
*See also individual names of health
    issues and hormones*
LDL, 61–63
lemon water, 47
LH (luteinizing hormone), 138
licorice root, 205
life expectancy, 14
lifestyle, 26, 57–58, 79–80
    after breast cancer, 166–167
    diet and, 59–67
    environmental pollutants and, 78–79
    foods and estrogen metabolism, 67–78
    importance of good health and, 58–59
    progesterone and, 132
light, sleep and, 224, 226, 230–231
lignans, 70–71
lipoic acid, 74
lipotropic complex, 128–129
liver
    caffeine and, 76
    healthy metabolism of, 46–47
    liver meridian, 43–46
    nutrients, 128–129
    Phase 1 metabolism, 48, 49–50
    Phase 2 metabolism, 48, 50–51

magnesium
    deficiency, 184
    glycinate, 212
    lab testing of, 190
    progesterone and, 131
mammograms, 146
marijuana, 225–226
measurement. *See* lab testing
medroxyprogesterone, 19, 120, 147–148
melatonin, 25, 89–90, 91, 219–220
    activation, 224
    case example, 229
    decline in, 221–222
    diet and, 225–227
    function, 222–223

high levels, 253
importance of good sleep, 220–221
insomnia and, 231
interactions with, 230
jet lag and, 230
measurement, 224–225
mood and, 94–95
premature aging and, 97
production of, 223–224
recreational drugs and, 225–227
Seasonal Affective Disorder and, 223,
    230–231
sleep problems, 221–222
substances that lower, 232
symptoms of low levels, 249
usage, 227–229
men
    andropause in, 15
    estrogen and, 151
    progesterone and, 127
menopause, 16, 143–144
    estrogen use and, 155–156,
        157–160
    health changes during, 146
    symptoms of, 82–83
    transitioning into, 145–146
    WHI study and, 34
    See also perimenopause
menstruation
    cycle length, and timing of
        progesterone, 124–125
    estrogen use and, 154–155
    lab testing during, 103, 104
    skipped cycles and estrogen, 145
    See also menopause; perimenopause
meridians
    change in, 83–84
    defined, 43–44
    liver meridian, 43–46
metabolites, 104
    See also DHEA
        (dehydroepiandrosterone)
methylation, 50–51
milk thistle, 128–129
Million Women Study, 33, 35
minerals, 26
    tests for deficiencies, 104
    for thyroid support, 212
mood problems, as symptom, 93–95

NAC (N-acetylcysteine), 74
natural hormones, 7
"naturalist" physicians, 1
"natural," safety and, 38
NeuroScience, 107
neurotransmitters, 93
New England Journal of Medicine, 234
nicotine, 226
"night owl" behavior, 224, 231
norepinephrine, 93
Nurses' Health Study (NHS), 32–33, 35,
    36–37
    dietary fat, 63
    lifestyle and, 59

omega-3/6 fatty acids, 64–66, 129–130
oral estrogen 31, 147–148
oral progesterone, 124–126
oral testosterone, 174
orgasm, 98
ovaries
    aging of, 137–138
    and hormonal ups and downs,
        142–143
    hysterectomy and, 160–161

Pap smears, 146
patches
    estrogen, 150
    testosterone, 174
pathways, 50
perimenopause, 15–16, 29
    estrogen use and, 154–155, 158–160
    low estrogen in, 144–145
    progesterone for, 115–116
    symptoms of, 82–83, 118–119,
        122–123, 132, 246
    See also menopause
pesticides, 78–79
phytoestrogens, 69–72
phytosterols, 72–73
Pierce Apothecary, 112
pineal gland, 222
plants, hormones derived from, 37–38
plastics, 78–79
PMS
    cases of, 132–135
    low progesterone and, 122–123
    symptoms, 87–88

treatments for, 128–131
polymorphic genetic testing, 53–55, 243
porcine extract, 206
prednisone, 192, 200. *See also* cortisol
pregnenolone, 197
    cascade, 191
    fatigue and, 92
    high, 252
    low, 248
    measuring, 197
    usage, 204
Premarin, 7–8, 33–35, 118
Prempro, 33–35
prescription drugs, 81–82
    antidepressants, 93–95, 143–144
    interference with thyroid activation, 185
    melatonin lowered by, 232
    sleeping pills, 222
    T4 activation and, 185
    See also individual names of hormones
probiotics, 52–53
progesterone, 24–25, 131–135
    after hysterectomy, 163
    for breast cancer, 37
    case examples, 157–160, 161–163
    confusion about, 120–121
    dosages for, 123–124
    early perimenopause and PMS,
        122–123
    herbal and vitamin supports for,
        127–131
    low levels of, 119–121
    measuring, 103, 104
    mood and, 95
    natural, 39, 121
    perimenopausal symptoms and,
        115–116, 118–119, 132, 246
    premature aging and, 96
    preparations, 123–127
    sleep and, 89, 91
    synthetic, 19, 31, 167
    timing for usage, 123, 124–125
    unbalanced, 117–118
    See also estrogen
Provera, 19, 33–35

qi, 3, 44–46
Quest Diagnostics, 107
quinones, 42

RBC magnesium test, 190
rebound sleep phase insomnia, 231
recreational drugs, melatonin and, 225–227
research studies
    on bioidentical hormones, 39, 121, 156
    safety and, 30–35
Rhein Consulting Laboratories, 107
rhemania, 207–208
rhodiola, 207
ring inserts, vaginal, 152

safety, 29–30
    bioidentical hormones and, 37–39
    estrogen use and, 54–55, 147–148, 156
    of growth hormone injections, 240
    major research studies and, 30–35, 156
    melatonin interactions, 230
    "natural" and, 38
    timing of hormones, 35–37
    See also hormone metabolism
salivary cortisol, 196
saliva tests, 102, 103, 105. See also lab testing
SAMe (S Adenosyl methionine), 94–95
saw palmetto, 171, 173
Seasonal Affective Disorder (SAD), 223, 230–231
selenium, 74
serotonin, 93
    low estradiol and, 143–144
    melatonin and, 223–224
sex drive, as symptom, 98
sex hormone binding globulin (SHBG), 101
sex hormones, supporting, 24–25. See also estrogen; progesterone; testosterone
shedding, of hair, 171
Shou Wu Wan, 173
Siberian ginseng, 207
side effects. See individual names of hormones
sitosterols, 72–73
16-hydroxyestrone (16-OH estrone), 41–42

sleep hormones, 219–220
    diet and, 225–227
    importance of good sleep, 220–222
    insomnia and, 231
    jet lag and, 230
    melatonin, 25, 89–90, 91, 94–95, 97, 222–232, 249
    mood and, 94–95
    premature aging and, 97
    Seasonal Affective Disorder and, 223, 230–231
    stages of sleep, 220–222, 226, 231
    as symptom, 84, 88–91
    symptoms of low levels, 249
somatomedins, 235
soy, 69–70
Spectracell Laboratories, 107
stages, of sleep, 220–222, 226, 231
statins, 62
stimulation test, cortisol, 197
stress, 192. See also cortisol
symptoms, 81–83, 86–88
    awareness of, 2, 3, 5, 21–22, 84–86, 241–243
    case example, 87–88
    Chinese perspective on, 83–84
    of excess hormones, 251–253
    of hypoadrenia, 180–182
    low energy as, 84, 91–93
    of low estrogen, 117, 143–145
    of low progesterone, 117, 119–120
    of low testosterone, 168
    of low hormones, 245–250
    low sex drive as, 98
    of low thyroid function, 181–182
    mood problems as, 93–95
    poor sleep as, 84, 88–91
    progesterone and, 118–119, 132
    showing age as, 95–97
    "symptom swapping," 6–7

targeted amino acid therapies, 165
taurine, 212
testosterone
    DHT, 170–171, 252
    estrogen conversion, 169
    hair loss and, 171–173
    high levels of, 173, 251–252
    low, 168, 247

measuring, 103, 169–170
side effects of, 170–171
in women, 168
See also estrogen
tests. *See* lab testing
thyroid hormones, 177–178
    adrenal extract sources and, 206
    adrenal glands and, 179–180, 190–198
    case examples, 213–218
    common problems, 178–179
    diet and, 211–213
    fatigue and, 93
    functional low thyroid, 183–185
    high, 252–253
    hypoadrenia and, 180–182
    iodine and, 183, 186–188
    low, 181–182, 248
    measuring, 23–24, 103, 188–190
    mood and, 95
    natural thyroid extract, 209–210
    normal thyroid gland function, 182–183
    premature aging and, 96, 97
    sex drive and, 98
    sleep and, 90, 91
    supporting, with bioidentical
        hormones, 25, 199–206, 208–218
    supporting, with herbs and vitamins,
        207–208, 211–213
    thyroid antibodies, 185–186
    TSH, defined, 182. *See also* TSH
        (thyroid-stimulating hormone)
    See also adrenal hormones
Thyrolar, 210
transdermal preparations
    estradiol, 39, 40
    progesterone, 123–126
    testosterone, 173–174
Trans-d Tropin (Trans-d), 237–239
TSH (thyroid-stimulating hormone),
    182–183
    blood test, 188–189
    diet and, 211–213
    response to therapy, 210–211
    T3, T4 forms, 183–185, 189–190
    thyroid hormone support and, 208–209
    See also thyroid hormones
24-hour urine tests, 46, 102, 104–105
    for aldosterone, 198

for cortisol, 196–197
for DHEA, 198
for growth hormone, 236
for thyroid, 189–190
2-methoxyestrone (2-ME estrone), 41, 55
tyrosine, 206, 212

University Compounding Pharmacy, 113
urinary frequency, 151–152
urine tests. *See* lab testing; 24-hour urine
    tests
uterine cancer, 148
uterus, hysterectomy and, 160–163

vaginal bleeding, abnormal, 124–125, 151
vaginal preparations
    estrogen, 151–160
    progesterone, 126–127
    vitamin E suppositories, 165
vaginitis, 151
vegetables
    antioxidants in, 73–74
    cruciferous, 67–69
    See also diet
vitamins, 26
    for adrenal support, 208
    antioxidants in, 74
    B, 129
    C, 74, 208
    D, 104
    E, 74, 130–131, 165
    for progesterone support, 127–131
    for thyroid support, 208, 211–213
vulvar testosterone, 174

wild yam, 126
Women's Health Initiative (WHI) study,
    4–5, 33–35
    age of subjects, 157
    dietary fat and, 63–64
    fear of hormones and, 18, 19
    on hormone support duration, 156
    lifestyle and, 59
Women's International Pharmacy, 113

yin deficiency, 8–9, 83–84, 179

zinc, 171, 173

1/12/16
0

615.36   Cohan, Phuli.
C
         The natural hormone
         makeover.

DATE			